The Fastest Anti-Inflammatory Cookbook

Easy and Delicious Cookbook to Create Your Meals in Minutes

Thomas Jollif

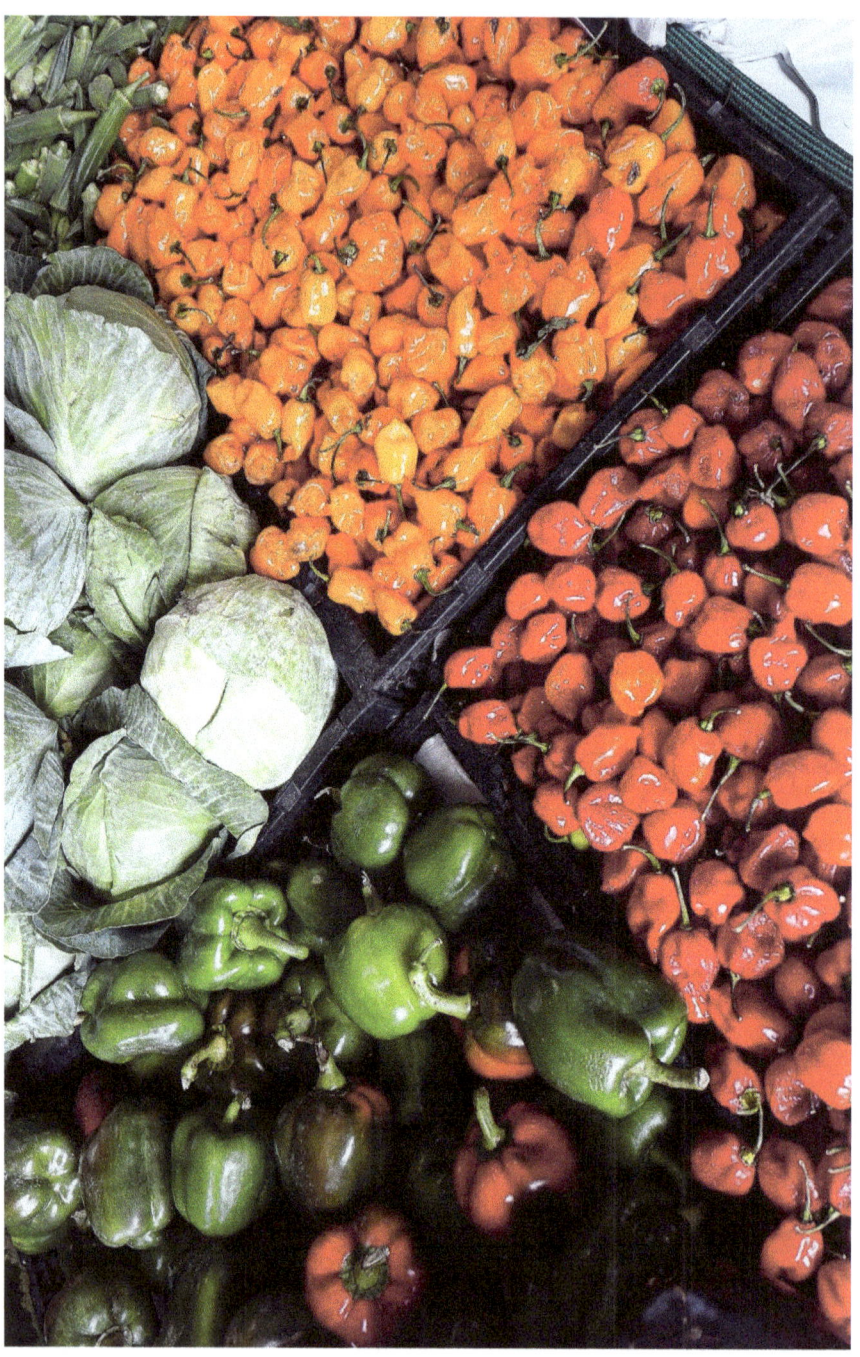

© copyright 2021 – all rights reserved.

the content contained within this book may not be reproduced, duplicated or transmitted without direct written permission from the author or the publisher.

under no circumstances will any blame or legal responsibility be held against the publisher, or author, for any damages, reparation, or monetary loss due to the information contained within this book. either directly or indirectly.

legal notice:

this book is copyright protected. this book is only for personal use. you cannot amend, distribute, sell, use, quote or paraphrase any part, or the content within this book, without the consent of the author or publisher.

disclaimer notice:

please note the information contained within this document is for educational and entertainment purposes only. all effort has been executed to present accurate, up to date, and reliable, complete information. no warranties of any kind are declared or implied. readers acknowledge that the author is not engaging in the rendering of legal, financial, medical or professional advice. the content within this book has been derived from various sources. please consult a licensed professional before attempting any techniques outlined in this book.

by reading this document, the reader agrees that under no circumstances is the author responsible for any losses, direct or indirect, which are incurred as a result of the use of information contained within this document, including, but not limited to, — errors, omissions, or inaccuracies.

Table of Contents

BREAKFASTS 7

Almond Mascarpone Dumplings.. 7
Almond Pancakes with Coconut Flakes 9
Almond Scones.. 12
Anti-Inflammatory Breakfast Frittata............................ 14
Apple Bread 16
Apple Bruschetta with Almonds and Blackberries 18
Apple Oatmeal... 20
Apple, Ginger, and Rhubarb Muffins................................ 21
Bake Apple Turnover... 24
Baked French Toast Casserole 26

SMOOTHIES AND DRINKS 28

Almond Blueberry Smoothie... 28
Almond Butter Smoothies 30
Apple Cinnamon Water 31
Baby Kale Pineapple Smoothie 32
Beet and Cherry Smoothie 34
Beet Smoothie 35
Berry Shrub 37
Blackberry & Ginger Milkshake..................................... 38

SIDES 40

BEET HUMMUS 40

BROCCOLI AND BLACK BEANS STIR FRY 42

CARAMELIZED PEARS AND ONIONS 44

CAULIFLOWER BROCCOLI MASH 46

CILANTRO AND AVOCADO PLATTER 48

SAUCES AND DRESSINGS 49

APPLE AND TOMATO DIPPING SAUCE 49

BALSAMIC VINAIGRETTE 51

SNACKS 53

ALMOND AND HONEY HOMEMADE BAR 53

ALMONDS AND BLUEBERRIES YOGURT SNACK 56

ANTI-INFLAMMATORY KEY LIME PIE 58

ANTS ON A LOG 60

APPLE CRISP 61

APPLE SAUCE TREAT 64

AVOCADO AND EGG SANDWICH 65

SOUPS AND STEWS 67

ANTI-INFLAMMATORY SPRING PEA SOUP 67

ANTI-INFLAMMATORY SWEET POTATO SOUP 69

BACON & CHEESE SOUP 71

BEEF AND VEGGIE SOUP 73

BROCCOLI CHEDDAR & BACON SOUP 75

BROCCOLI SOUP WITH GORGONZOLA CHEESE 77

BROWN RICE AND SHITAKE MISO SOUP WITH SCALLION 79

BUFFALO SAUCE AND TURKEY SOUP 81
BUTTERNUT SQUASH SOUP WITH SHRIMP 83
CANNELLINI BEAN SOUP 85

DESSERTS 87

ALMOND BUTTER BALLS VEGAN 87
ALMOND COOKIES 88
ANTI-INFLAMMATORY APRICOT SQUARES 90
APPLE FRITTERS 92
AVOCADO BROWNIES 94
AVOCADO CHIA PARFAIT 96
AVOCADO CHOCO CAKE 98
AVOCADO CHOCOLATE MOUSSE 100
BANANA & AVOCADO MOUSSE 102
BANANA BARS 104

BREAKFASTS

Almond Mascarpone Dumplings

Time To Prepare: ten minutes
Time to Cook: ten minutes
Yield: Servings 6

Ingredients:

- ¼ cup ground almonds
- ¼ cup honey
- 1 cup all-purpose unbleached flour
- 1 cup whole-wheat flour
- 1 tablespoon butter
- 1 teaspoon extra-virgin olive oil
- 2 teaspoons apple juice
- 3 ounces mascarpone cheese
- 4 egg whites

Directions:

1. Strain together both types of flour in a big container. Stir in the almonds.
2. In a different container, whisk together the egg whites, cheese, oil, and juice on moderate speed using an electric mixer.

3. Place the flour, and egg white mixture with a dough hook on moderate speed or using your hands until a dough forms.
4. Boil 1 gallon water in a medium-size saucepot. Take a scoop of dough and use a second spoon to push it into the boiling water. Cook up to the dumpling floats to the top, minimum 5 to ten minutes. You can cook several dumplings at once — just take care not to crowd the pot.
5. Take off using a slotted spoon and drain using paper towels.
6. Warm a medium-size sauté pan on moderate to high heat.
7. Put in the butter, then put the dumplings in the pan and cook until light brown.
8. Set on serving plates and sprinkle with honey.

Nutritional Info: Calories: 254 ‖ Fat: 6.4 g ‖ Protein: 7 g ‖ Sodium: 20 mg ‖ Fiber: 3.5 g ‖ Carbohydrates: 44 g

Almond Pancakes with Coconut Flakes

Time To Prepare: 5 minutes
Time to Cook: ten minutes
Yield: Servings 6

Ingredients:

- ¼ cup coconut flakes, sweetened
- ¼ cup of water
- ¼ tsp. coconut oil
- ½ cup unsweetened applesauce
- 1 cup almond flour, finely milled
- 1 overripe banana, mashed
- 2 eggs, yolks, and whites separated
- 2 Tbsp. blanched almond flakes
- Dash of cinnamon powder
- Garnish
- Pinch of sea salt
- Pure maple syrup, use sparingly

Directions:

1. Whisk egg whites until tender peaks form.
2. Except for egg whites and coconut oil, mix rest of the ingredients in a different container. Mix until batter comes together.

3. Lightly fold in egg whites. Ensure that you do not over mix, or the pancake will become dense and chewy.
4. Pour oil into a nonstick frying pan set on moderate heat.
5. Wait for the oil to heat up before dropping in roughly ½ cup of batter. Cook until each side are set, and bubbles form in the middle. Turn on the other side then cook for an extra two minutes.
6. Move flapjacks to a plate. Repeat step until all batter is cooked. Pour in more oil into the frying pan only if required. This recipe should yield between four to 6 moderate-sized pancakes.
7. Stack pancakes. Pour the desired amount of pure maple syrup on top. Decorate each stack with cinnamon-flavored almond-coconut flakes just before you serve.
8. For the decorate, set the oven to 350°F for minimum ten minutes before use. Coat a baking sheet using parchment paper. Set aside.
9. Mix almond and coconut flakes together in a container. Spread mixture uniformly on a readied baking sheet.
10. Bake for 7 to ten minutes until flakes turn golden brown. Stir almond and coconut flakes once midway through roasting to stop over-browning.
11. Take away the baking sheet from the oven. Cool almond and coconut flakes for minimum ten minutes before drizzling in cinnamon powder and salt. Toss to blend. Set aside.

Nutritional Info: Calories: 62 kcal ‖ Protein: 2.24 g ‖ Fat: 4.01 g ‖ Carbohydrates: 4.46 g

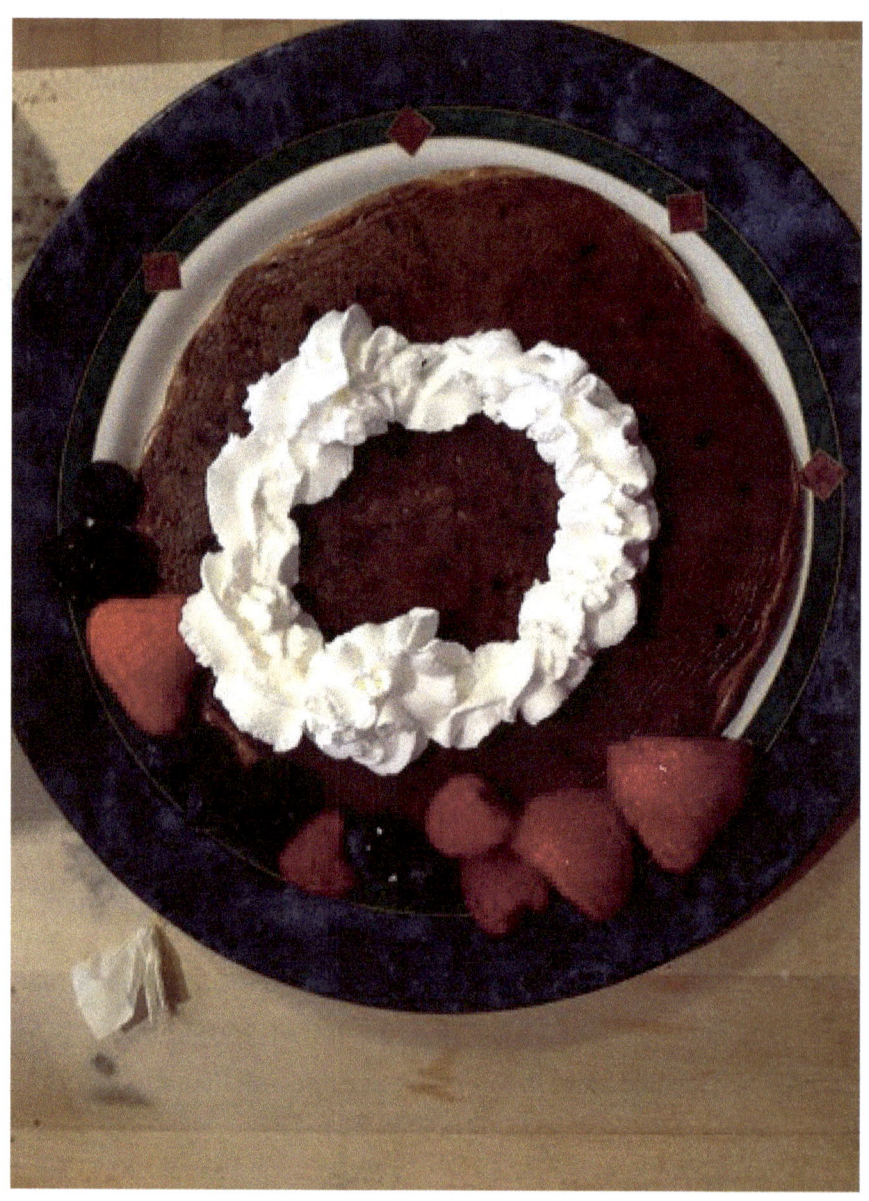

Almond Scones

Time To Prepare: ten minutes
Time to Cook: twenty minutes
Yield: Servings 6

Ingredients:
- 1 cup almonds
- ¼ cup arrowroot flour
- 1 tablespoon coconut flour
- 1 teaspoon ground turmeric
- Salt, to taste
- Freshly ground black pepper, to taste
- 1 egg
- ¼ cup essential olive oil
- 3 tablespoons raw honey
- 1 teaspoon vanilla flavoring
- 1 1/3 cups almond flour

Directions:
1. In a mixer, put almonds then pulse till chopped roughly
2. Move the chopped almonds in a big container.
3. Put flours and spices and mix thoroughly.
4. In another container, put the rest of the ingredients and beat till well blended.
5. Place the flour mixture into the egg mixture then mix till well blended.

6. Position a plastic wrap over the cutting board.
7. Put the dough over the cutting board.
8. Use both your hands to pat into 1-inch thick circle.
9. Chop the circle in 6 wedges.
10. Set the scones onto a cookie sheet in a single layer.
11. Bake for minimum fifteen-20 minutes.

Nutritional Info: Calories: 304 ‖ Fat: 3g ‖ Carbohydrates: 22g ‖ Fiber: 6g ‖ Protein: 20g

Anti-Inflammatory Breakfast Frittata

Time To Prepare: ten minutes
Time to Cook: forty minutes
Yield: Servings 4

Ingredients:

- ¼ cup water
- ½ tsp. cracked black pepper
- ½ tsp. ground turmeric
- 1 onion, chopped
- 1 tbsp. minced garlic
- 125g firm tofu
- 4 big eggs
- 450g baby spinach
- 450g button mushrooms
- 6 egg whites
- Kosher salt to taste

Directions:

1. Set the oven to 350F.
2. Sauté the mushrooms in a little bit of extra virgin olive oil in a big non-stick ovenproof pan on moderate heat. Put in the onions once the mushrooms start turning golden and

cook for about three minutes until the onions become tender.

3. Mix in the garlic then cook for minimum half a minute until aromatic before you put in the spinach. Pour in water, cover, and cook until the spinach becomes wilted for approximately 2 minutes.
4. Take off the lid and carry on cooking up to the water evaporates. Now, mix the eggs, egg whites, tofu, pepper, turmeric, and salt in a container. When all the liquid has vaporized, pour in the egg mixture, allow to cook for approximately 2 minutes until the edges start setting, then move to the oven and bake for approximately twenty-five minutes or until cooked.
5. Remove from the oven then allow it to sit for minimum five minutes before cutting it into four equivalent portions and serving.
6. Enjoy!

Nutritional Info: Calories: 521 kcal ‖ Protein: 29.13 g ‖ Fat: 10.45 g ‖ Carbohydrates: 94.94 g

Apple Bread

Time To Prepare: twenty-five minutes
Time to Cook: 1 hour and ten minutes
Yield: Servings 8

Ingredients:

- ¼ tsp. baking powder
- 1 cup peeled, chopped apples
- 1 packet yeast
- 1 tbsp. cinnamon mixed with 1 tablespoon sugar
- 1 tsp. Salt
- 1¾ cups all-purpose flour
- 1¾ cups whole-wheat flour
- 1 1/3 cups warm water
- 3 tbsp. sugar
- 3 tbsp. tender butter

Directions:

1. Mix yeast, ½ teaspoon sugar, and 1/3 cup water in a container. Allow to sit for five minutes.
2. In a mixing container, put together remaining water, butter, remaining sugar, salt, and baking powder then mix.
3. Mix in the all-purpose flour, then the yeast mixture using an electric mixer. Place the whole-wheat flour. Knead the dough hook for minimum ten minutes.
4. Place the dough into an oiled container.

5. Cover then rises in a warm place for minimum a couple of hours until doubled in bulk.
6. Punch down dough, then form into a rectangle.
7. Spread the apples on the dough and dust with the cinnamon sugar.
8. Roll into a cylinder and put in an oiled loaf pan. Cover and allow it to rise in a warm for 90 minutes until doubled in size.
9. Preheat your oven to 350°F. Uncover bread and bake for about fifty minutes.

Nutritional Info: Calories: 258 ‖ Fat: 5 g ‖ Protein: 7 g ‖ Sodium: 294 mg ‖ Fiber: 4.5 g ‖ Carbohydrates: 48 g

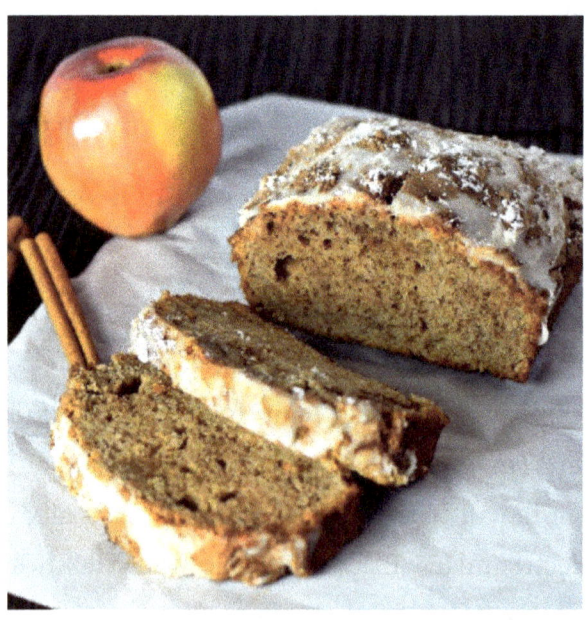

Apple Bruschetta with Almonds and Blackberries

Time To Prepare: twenty minutes
Time to Cook: thirty minutes
Yield: Servings 5

Ingredients:

- ¼ cup blackberries, thawed, lightly mashed
- ½ tsp. fresh lemon juice
- 1 apple, cut into ¼-inch thick half-moons
- 1/8 cup almond slivers, toasted
- Sea salt

Directions:

1. Sprinkle lemon juice on apple slices. Place these on a tray coated with parchment paper.
2. Spread a small number of mashed berries on top of each slice. Top these off with the desired amount of almond slivers.
3. Drizzle sea salt on "bruschetta" just before you serve.

Nutritional Info: Calories: 56 kcal ‖ Protein: 1.53 g ‖ Fat: 1.43 g ‖ Carbohydrates: 9.87 g

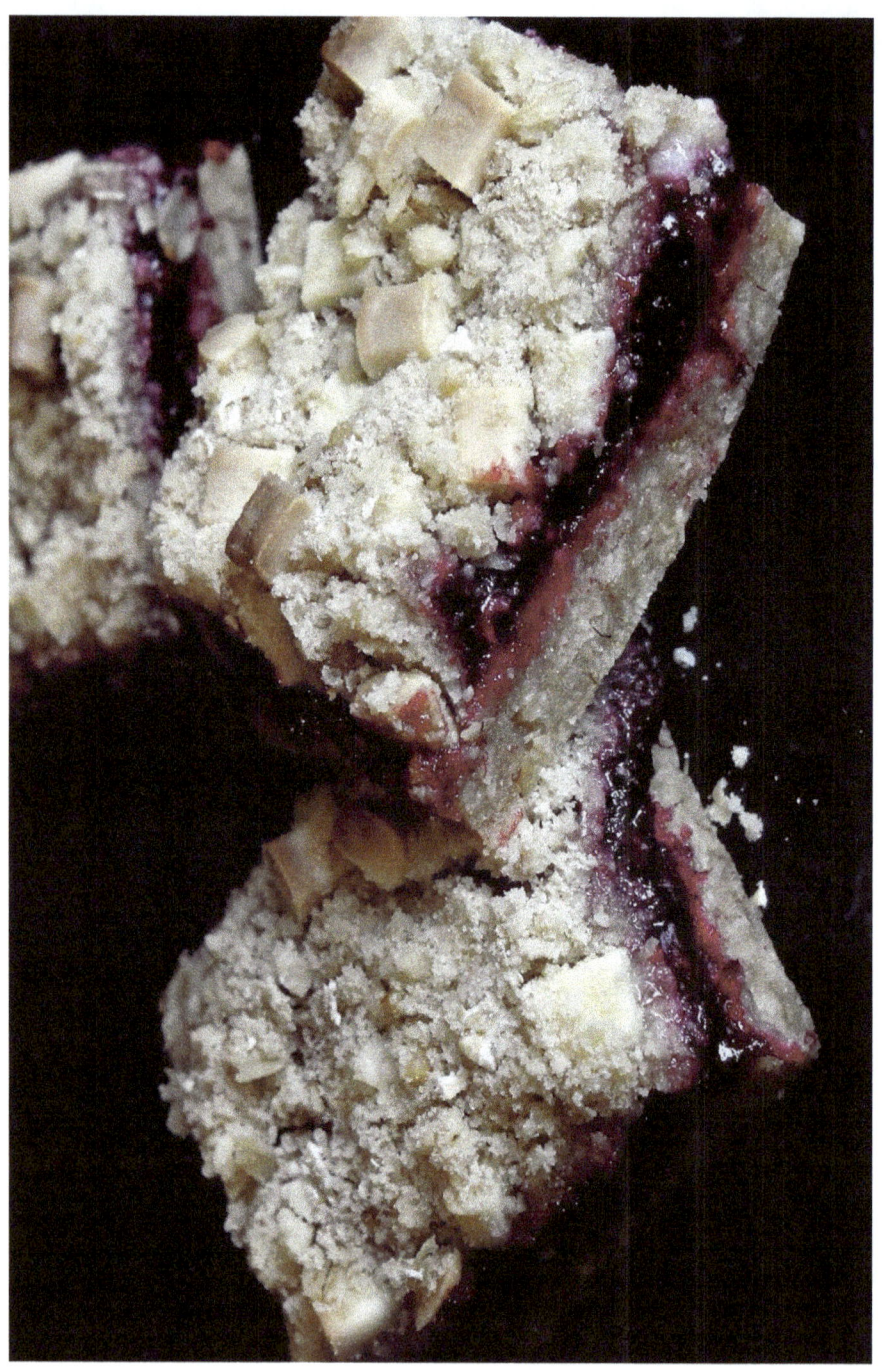

Apple Oatmeal

Time To Prepare: ten minutes
Time to Cook: five minutes
Yield: Servings 2

Ingredients:
- ¼ cup fresh apple juice
- 1 chopped apple, (unpeeled or peeled)
- 1 cup of any non-fat milk, coconut milk or almond milk (not necessary)
- 1 cup water
- 1 teaspoon ground cinnamon
- 2/3 cups rolled oats

Directions:
1. Put the water, juice, and the apple in a deep pot. Bring to boil on moderate heat.
2. Put in the oats and cinnamon. Bring to another boil. Reduce the heat temperature and allow it to simmer for about three minutes or until it is thick.
3. Split the serving into two and serve with milk.

Nutritional Info: Calories: 277 kcal ‖ Protein: 12.69 g ‖ Fat: 7.69 g ‖ Carbohydrates: 52.71 g

Apple, Ginger, and Rhubarb Muffins

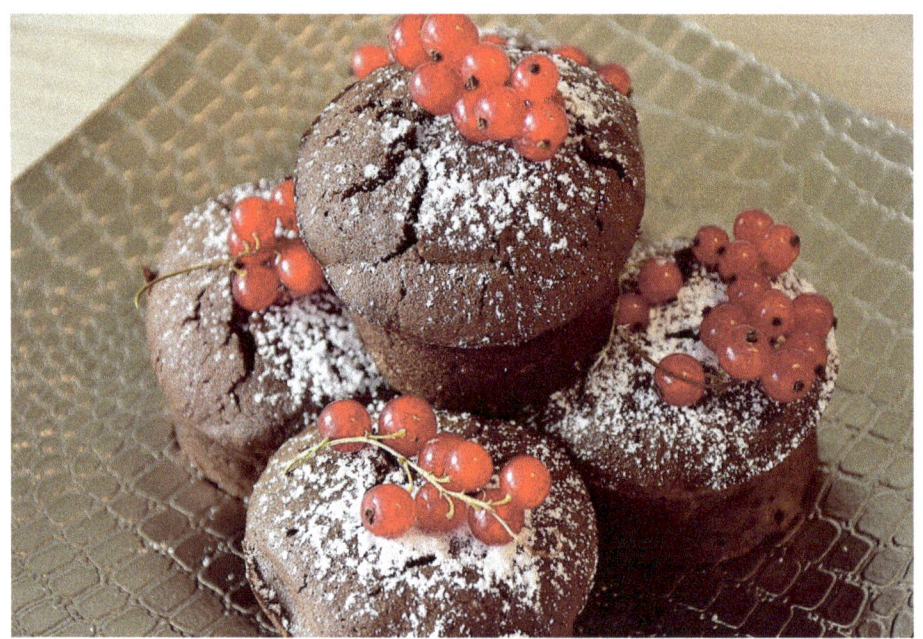

Time To Prepare: fifteen minutes
Time to Cook: twenty-five minutes
Yield: Servings 4

Ingredients:

- ¼ cup brown rice flour
- ¼ cup extra virgin olive oil

- ½ cup buckwheat flour
- ½ cup thoroughly ground almonds
- ½ tsp. ground cinnamon
- ½ tsp. ground ginger
- 1 big egg
- 1 cup finely chopped rhubarb
- 1 small apple, peeled and finely diced
- 1 tbsp. linseed meal
- 1 tsp. pure vanilla extract
- 1/3 cup almond/ rice milk
- 1/8 cup unrefined raw sugar
- 2 tbsp. arrowroot flour
- 2 tbsp. crystallized ginger, finely chopped
- 2 tsp. gluten-free baking powder
- A pinch of fine sea salt

Directions:

1. Set the oven to 350F grease an eight-cup muffin tin and line with paper cases.
2. Mix the almond four, linseed meal, ginger and sugar in a mixing container. Sieve this mixture over the other flours, spices and baking powder and use a whisk to blend well.
3. Mix in the apple and rhubarb in the flour mixture until uniformly coated.
4. In a different container, whisk the milk, vanilla, and egg then pour it into the dry mixture. Stir until just blended – do not overwork the batter as this can yield very tough muffins.

5. Scoop the mixture into the position muffin tin and top with a few slices of rhubarb. Bake for minimum twenty-five minutes, till they start turning golden or when an inserted toothpick emerges clean.
6. Remove from the oven and allow it to sit for minimum five minutes before transferring the muffins to a wire rack for further cooling.
7. Serve warm with a glass of squeezed juice.
8. Enjoy!

Nutritional Info: Calories: 325 kcal ‖ Protein: 6.32 g ‖ Fat: 9.82 g ‖ Carbohydrates: 55.71 g

Bake Apple Turnover

Time To Prepare: thirty minutes
Time to Cook: twenty-five minutes
Yield: Servings 4

Ingredients:

- ½ cup palm sugar, crumbled using your hands to loosen granules
- ½ tsp. cinnamon powder
- 1 egg white, whisked in
- 1 frozen puff pastry, thawed
- 1 Tbsp. almond flour
- 2 Tbsp. water
- 4 apples, peeled, cored, diced into bite-sized pieces
- All-purpose flour, for rolling out the dough
- For the egg wash
- For the turnovers

Directions:

1. To make the filling: mix almond flour, cinnamon powder, and palm sugar until these resemble coarse meal. Toss in diced apples until thoroughly coated. Set aside.
2. On a mildly floured surface, roll the puff pastry until ¼ inch thin. Cut into 8 pieces of 4" x 4" squares.

3. Split prepared apples into 8 equivalent portions. Ladle on individual puff pastry squares. Fold in half diagonally. Push edges to secure.
4. Put each filled pastry on a baking tray coated with parchment paper. Make sure there is ample space between pastries.
5. Freeze for minimum twenty minutes, or till ready to bake.
6. Preheat your oven to 400°F or 205°C for at ten minutes.
7. Brush frozen pastries with egg wash. Bring in a hot oven, and cook for twelve to fifteen minutes, or until these turn golden brown all over.
8. Take off the baking tray in your oven instantly. Cool slightly for easier handling.
9. Put 1 apple turnover on a plate. Serve warm.

Nutritional Info: Calories: 203 kcal ∥ Protein: 5.29 g ∥ Fat: 4.4 g ∥ Carbohydrates: 38.25 g

Baked French Toast Casserole

Time To Prepare: twenty minutes
Time to Cook: forty-five minutes
Yield: Servings 12

Ingredients:

- ½ lb. blueberries
- ½ lb. raspberries
- ¾ cup strawberries
- 1 cup of egg white liquid
- 1 lb. French bread
- 1 teaspoon of vanilla extract
- 1/3 cup maple syrup
- 1½ cups of rice milk,
- 6 eggs

Directions:

1. Cut the bread into little cubes. Keep them in a greased casserole dish.
2. Put in all the berries. Only leave a few for the topping.
3. Mix together the egg whites, eggs, rice milk, and maple syrup in a container.
4. Mix well.
5. Place the egg mixture on the top of the bread. Push the bread down. All pieces must be soaked well.
6. Put in berries on the top. Fill up the holes, if any.

7. Place in your fridge covered for a couple of hours at least.
8. Take out the casserole half an hour before you bake.
9. Set the oven to 350 degrees F.
10. Now, bake your casserole uncovered for half an hour
11. Bake for another fifteen minutes covered with a foil.
12. Let it rest for 15 minutes.
13. Serve it warm with maple syrup.

Nutritional Info: Calories 200 ‖ Carbohydrates: 31g ‖ Cholesterol: 93mg ‖ Total Fat: 4g ‖ Protein: 10g ‖ Fiber: 2g ‖ Sodium: 288mg ‖ Sugar: 10g

Smoothies and Drinks

Almond Blueberry Smoothie

Time To Prepare: ten minutes
Time to Cook: 0 minutes
Yield: Servings 1

Ingredients:
- 1 banana
- 1 cup frozen blueberries
- 1 tbsp. almond butter
- 1/2 cup almond milk
- Water, as required

Directions:
1. Put in everything to a blender jug.
2. Cover the jug firmly.
3. Blend until the desired smoothness is achieved. Serve and enjoy!

Nutritional Info: Calories: 211 ∥ Fat: 0.2 g ∥ Protein: 5.6 g ∥ Carbohydrates: 3.4 g ∥ Fiber: 2.3 g

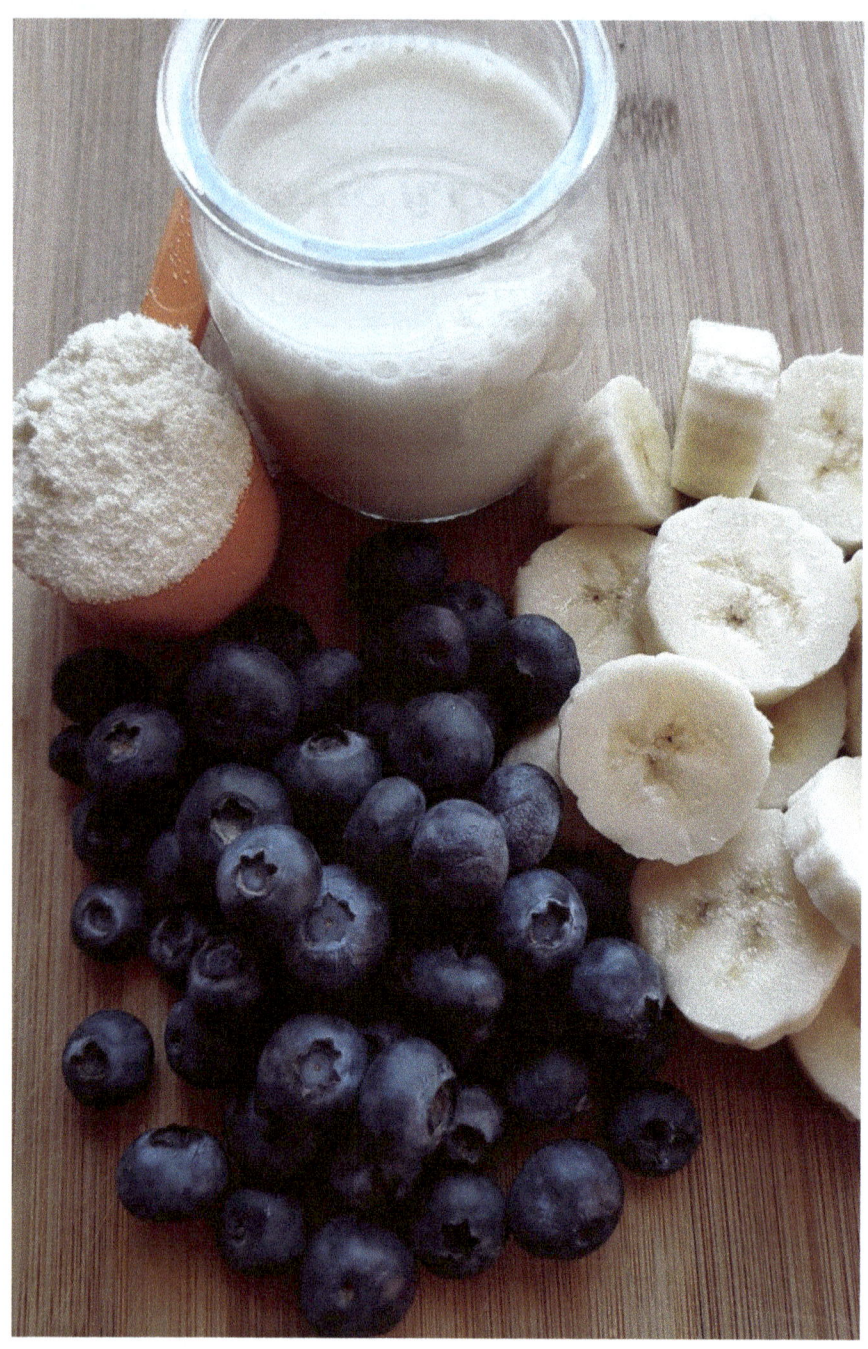

Almond Butter Smoothies

Time To Prepare: five minutes

Time to Cook: 0 minutes

Yield: Servings 1

Ingredients:

- 1 banana, if possible frozen for a creamier shake
- 1 cup of hemp milk
- 1 scoop of hemp protein
- 1 Tablespoon natural almond butter
- few ice cubes

Directions:

Blend all ingredients together and enjoy!

Nutritional Info: Calories: 533 kcal ‖ Protein: 31.23 g ‖ Fat: 26.31 g ‖ Carbohydrates: 47.13 g

Apple Cinnamon Water

Time To Prepare: five minutes
Time to Cook: five minutes
Yield: Servings 4

Ingredients:

- 1 whole apple, diced
- 5 cinnamon sticks
- Water to cover contents

Directions:

1. Put ingredients in the steamer basket. Put in pot.
2. Put in water cover contents.
3. Secure the lid. Cook on HIGH pressure five minutes.
4. When done, depressurize swiftly.
5. Remove steamer basket. Discard cooked produce.
6. Let flavored water cool. Chill completely before you serve.

Nutritional Info: Calories: 194 ‖ Fat: 0g ‖ Carbohydrates: 12g ‖ Protein: 0g

Baby Kale Pineapple Smoothie

Time To Prepare: five minutes
Time to Cook: 0 minutes
Yield: Servings 1

Ingredients:

- 1 cup almond milk
- 1 cup Kale
- 1 tablespoon hemp protein powder
- 1/2 cup frozen pineapple

Directions:

Put the almond milk, pineapple, and greens in the blender and blend until the desired smoothness is achieved.

Nutritional Info: Calories: 389 kcal ‖ Protein: 20.29 g ‖ Fat: 16.2 g ‖ Carbohydrates: 42.29 g

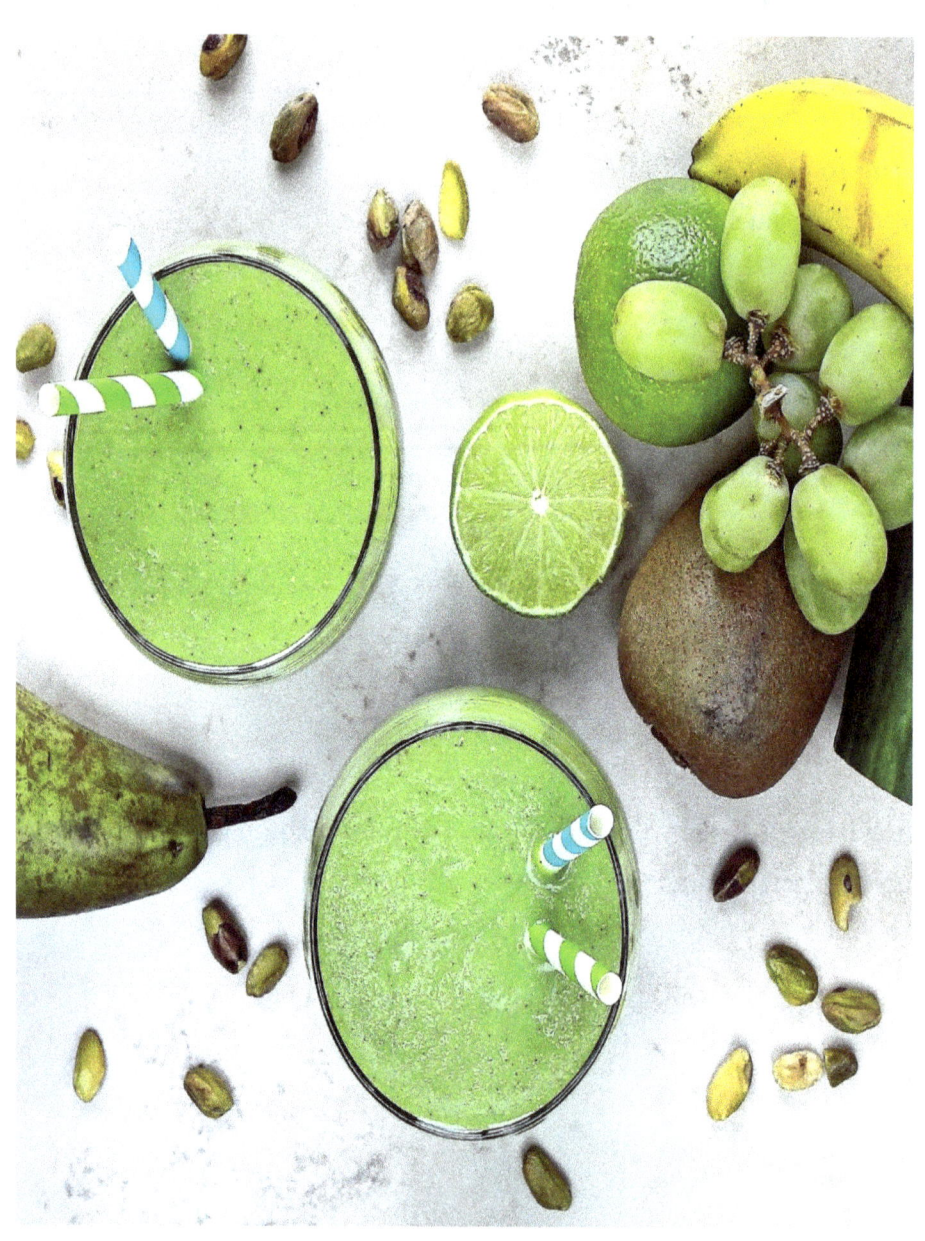

Beet and Cherry Smoothie

Time To Prepare: five minutes
Time to Cook: 0 minutes
Yield: Servings 4

Ingredients:

- ½ cup frozen cherries, pitted
- ½ teaspoon frozen banana
- 1 tablespoon almond butter
- 10-ounce almond milk, unsweetened
- 2 small beets, peeled and slice into four

Directions:

1. Put in all ingredients in a blender.
2. Blend until the desired smoothness is achieved.

Nutritional Info: Calories 470 ‖ Carbohydrates: 24 g ‖ Fat: 38 g ‖ Protein: 16 g

Beet Smoothie

Time To Prepare: ten minutes
Time to Cook: 0 minutes
Yield: Servings 2

Ingredients:

- 1 tbsp. almond butter
- 1/2 banana, peeled and frozen
- 1/2 cup cherries, pitted
- 10 oz. almond milk, unsweetened
- 2 beets, peeled and quartered

Directions:

1. In your blender, combine the milk with the beets, banana, cherries, and butter.
2. Pulse thoroughly, pour into glasses, before you serve. Enjoy!

Nutritional Info: Calories: 165 ‖ Fat: 5 g ‖ Protein: 5 g ‖ Carbohydrates: 22 g ‖ Fiber: 6 g

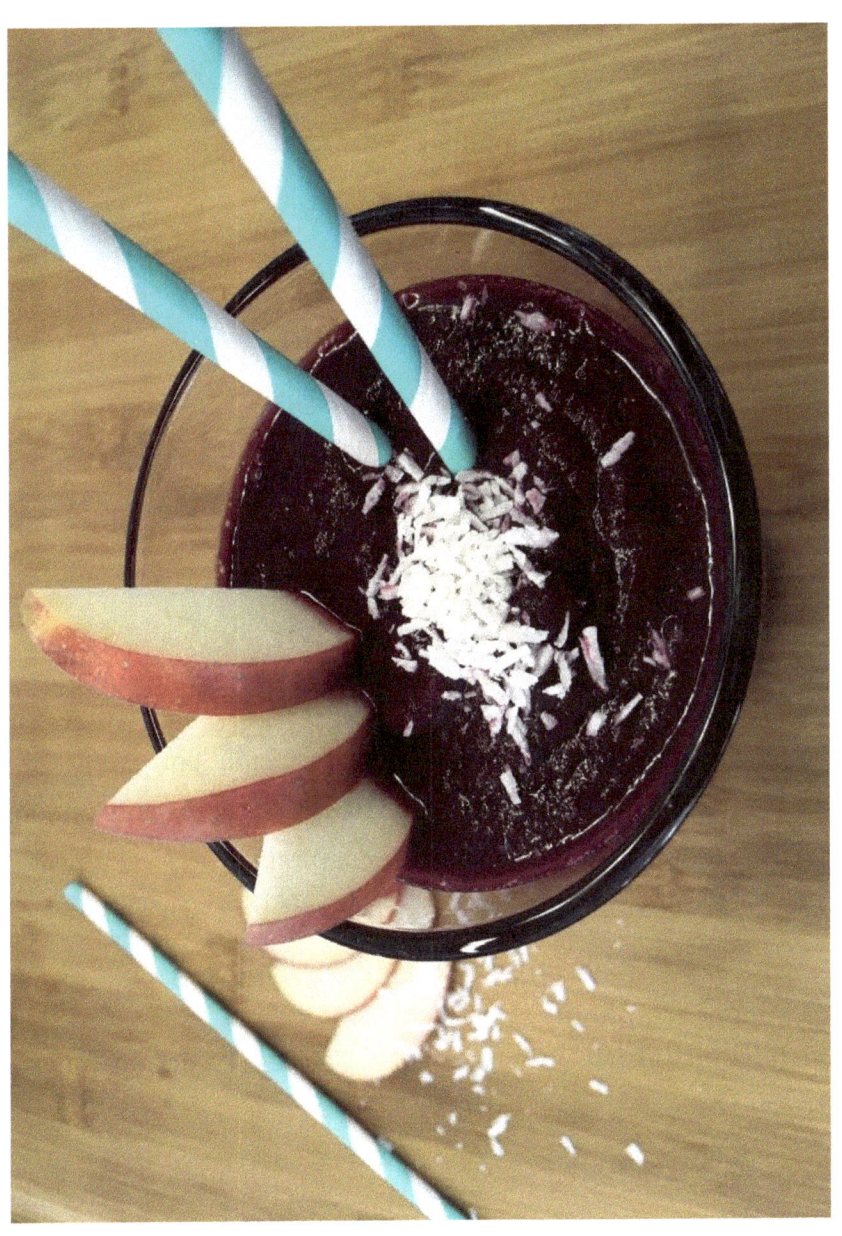

Berry Shrub

Time To Prepare: ten minutes
Time to Cook: twenty minutes
Yield: Servings 4

Ingredients:

- ½ a cup of chopped fresh oregano
- 1 cup of dried elderberries
- 2 cups of apple cider vinegar
- 2 cups of honey
- 2 cups of water

Directions:

1. Put in listed ingredients to the instant pot.
2. Secure the lid. Cook on HIGH pressure twenty minutes.
3. When done, depressurize naturally.
4. Pour ingredients through a sieve into a jar.
5. Let cool down. Chill.

Nutritional Info: Calories: 127 ‖ Fat: 0g ‖ Carbohydrates: 6g ‖ Protein: 0g

Blackberry & Ginger Milkshake

Time To Prepare: five minutes

Time to Cook: 0 minutes

Yield: Servings 2

Ingredients:

- 1 thumb-sized piece of ginger, grated
- 2 cups of almond milk
- 2 cups of blackberries, washed
- 2 cups of chopped peaches

Directions:

1. Combine all ingredients to a blender or juicer and blend until the desired smoothness is achieved.
2. Serve with a scattering of fresh blackberries and enjoy!

Nutritional Info: Calories: 619 kcal ‖ Protein: fifteen.42 g ‖ Fat: 11.63 g ‖ Carbohydrates: 123.04 g

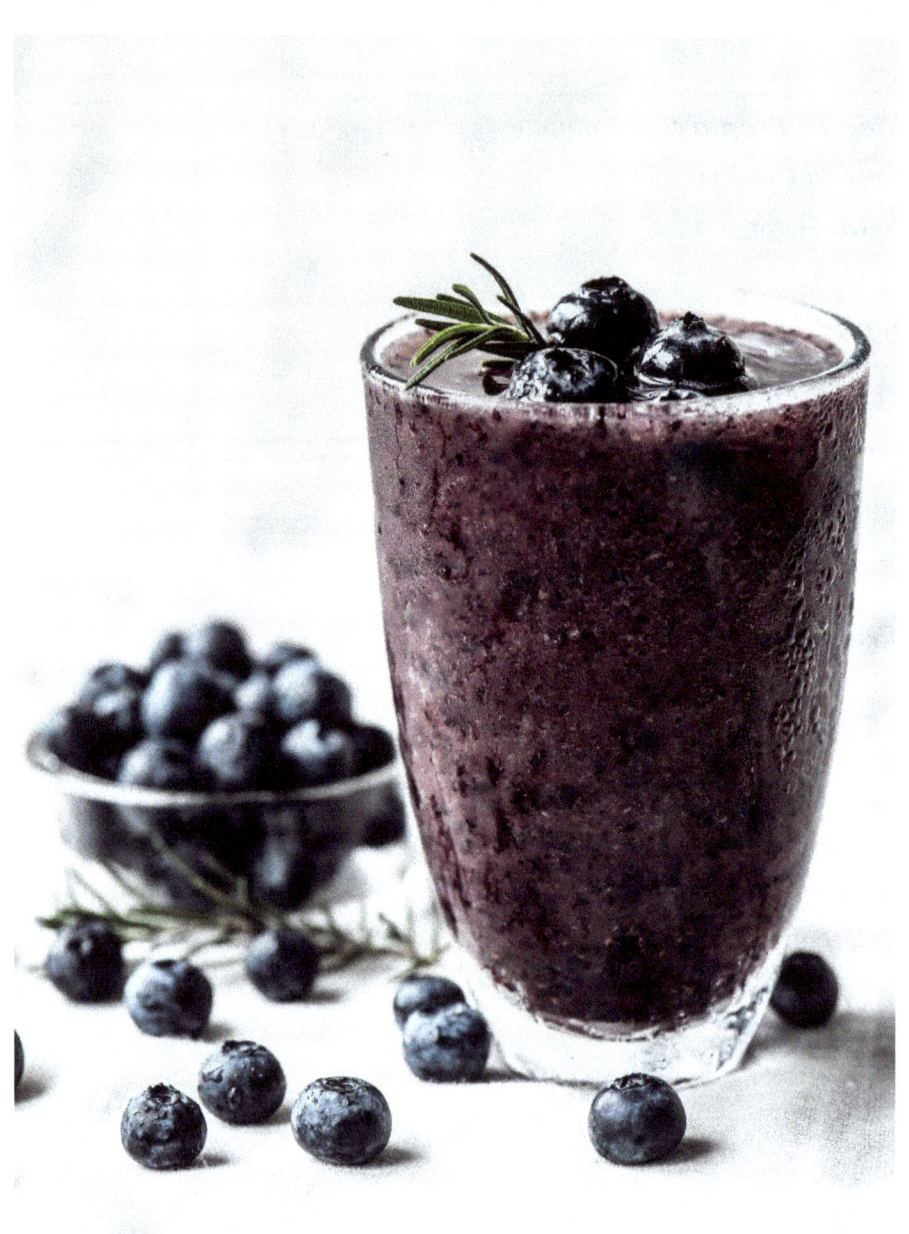

SIDES

Beet Hummus

Time To Prepare: five minutes
Time to Cook: 0 minutes
Yield: Servings 2

Ingredients:
- ¼ tsp of chili flakes
- ½ cup of olive oil
- ½ tsp of oregano
- ½ tsp of salt
- 1 ½ tsp of cumin
- 1 ¾ cup of chickpeas
- 1 clove of garlic
- 1 nub of fresh ginger
- 1 skinless roasted beet
- 1 tsp of curry
- 1 tsp of maple syrup
- 2 tbsp. of sunflower seeds
- Juice of one lemon

Directions:
1. Blend all together the ingredients in a food processor until they're smooth and decorate them with sunflower seeds.

2. Enjoy!

Nutritional Info: ‖ Calories: 423 kcal ‖ Protein: 13.98 g ‖ Fat: 24.26 g ‖ Carbohydrates: 40.13 g

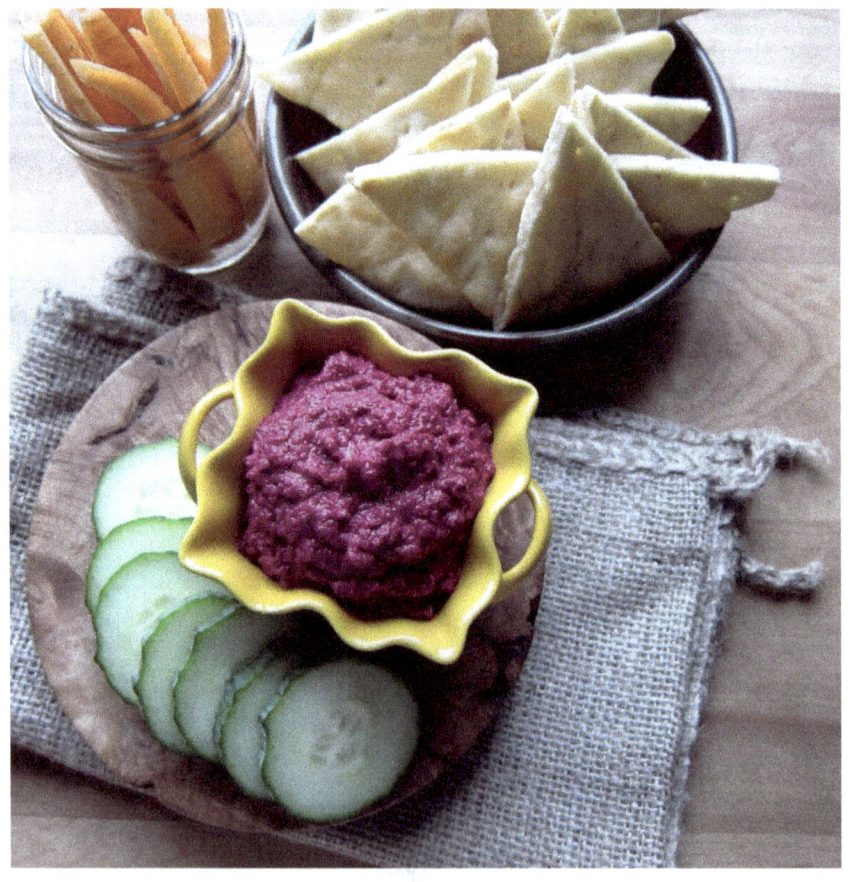

Broccoli and Black Beans Stir Fry

Time To Prepare: ten minutes
Time to Cook: fifteen minutes
Yield: Servings 4

Ingredients:

- 1 tablespoon sesame oil
- 2 cloves garlic, thoroughly minced
- 2 cups cooked black beans
- 2 teaspoons ginger, finely chopped
- 4 cups broccoli florets
- 4 teaspoons sesame seeds
- A big pinch red chili flakes
- A pinch turmeric powder
- Lime juice to taste (not necessary)
- Salt to taste

Directions:

1. Pour enough water to immerse the bottom of the deep cooking pan by an inch. Put a strainer on the deep cooking pan. Put broccoli florets on the strainer. Steam the broccoli for about six minutes.
2. Put a big frying pan on moderate heat. Put in sesame oil. When the oil is just warm, put in sesame seeds, chili flakes,

ginger, garlic, turmeric powder and salt. Sauté for about 2 minutes until aromatic.
3. Put in steamed broccoli and black beans and sauté until meticulously heated.
4. Put in lime juice and stir.
5. Serve hot.

Nutritional Info: ‖ Calories: 196 kcal ‖ Protein: 11.2 g ‖ Fat: 7.25 g ‖ Carbohydrates: 23.45 g

Caramelized Pears and Onions

Time To Prepare: five minutes
Time to Cook: thirty-five minutes
Yield: Servings 4

Ingredients:

- 1 tablespoon olive oil
- 2 firm red pears, cored and quartered
- 2 red onion, cut into wedges
- Salt and pepper, to taste

Directions:

1. Preheat the oven to 425 degrees F
2. Put the pears and onion on a baking tray
3. Sprinkle with olive oil
4. Sprinkle with salt and pepper
5. Bake using your oven for a little more than half an hour
6. Serve and enjoy!

Nutritional Info: ‖ Calories: 101 ‖ Fat: 4g ‖ Carbohydrates: 17g ‖ Protein: 1g

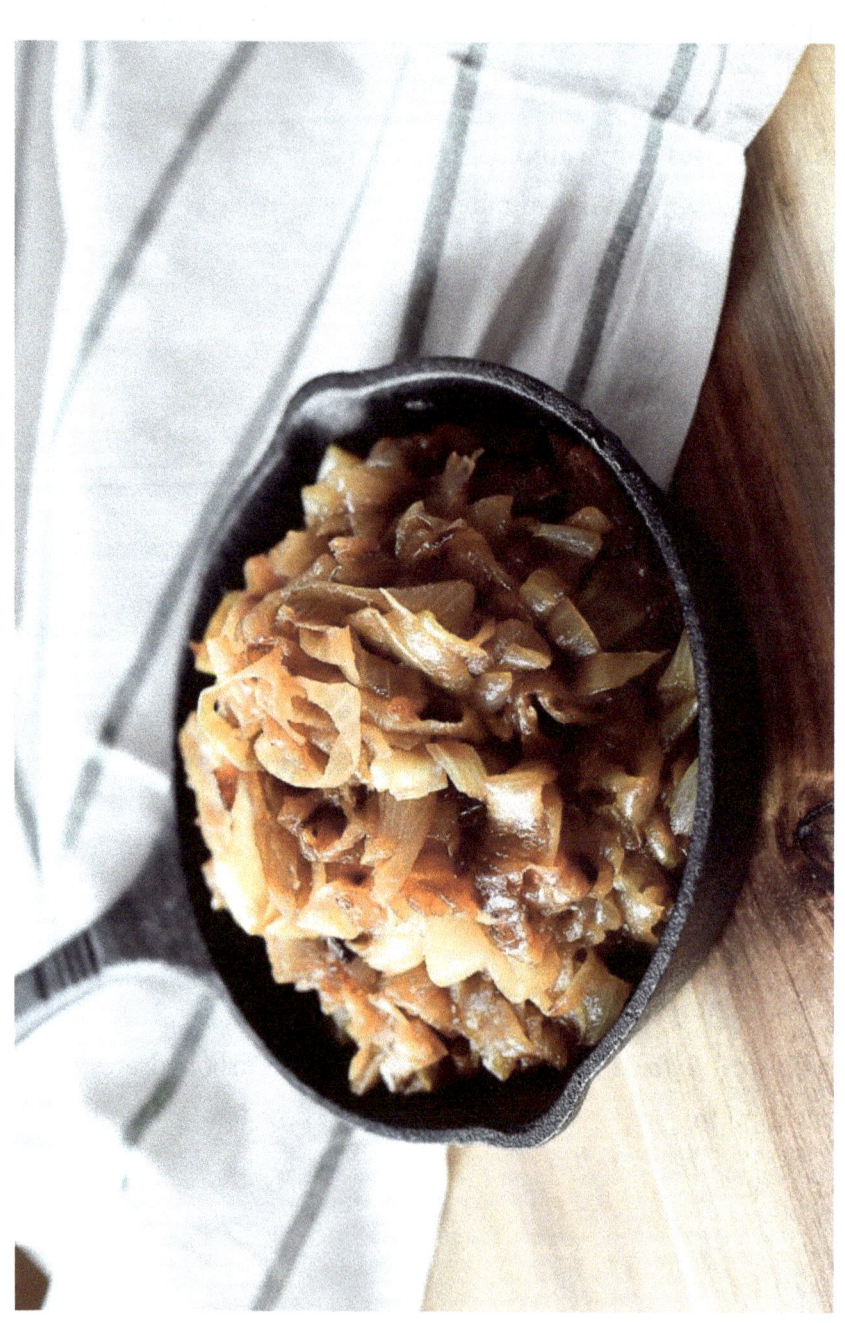

Cauliflower Broccoli Mash

Time To Prepare: five minutes
Time to Cook: ten minutes
Yield: Servings 6

Ingredients:

- 1 big head cauliflower, cut into chunks
- 1 small head broccoli, cut into florets
- 1 teaspoon salt
- 3 tablespoons extra virgin olive oil
- Pepper, to taste

Directions:

1. Take a pot and put in oil then heat it
2. Put in the cauliflower and broccoli
3. Sprinkle with salt and pepper to taste
4. Keep stirring to make vegetable soft
5. Put in water if required
6. When is already cooked, use a food processor or a potato masher to puree the vegetables
7. Serve and enjoy!

Nutritional Info: ‖ Calories: 39 ‖ Fat: 3g ‖ Carbohydrates: 2g ‖ Protein: 0.89g

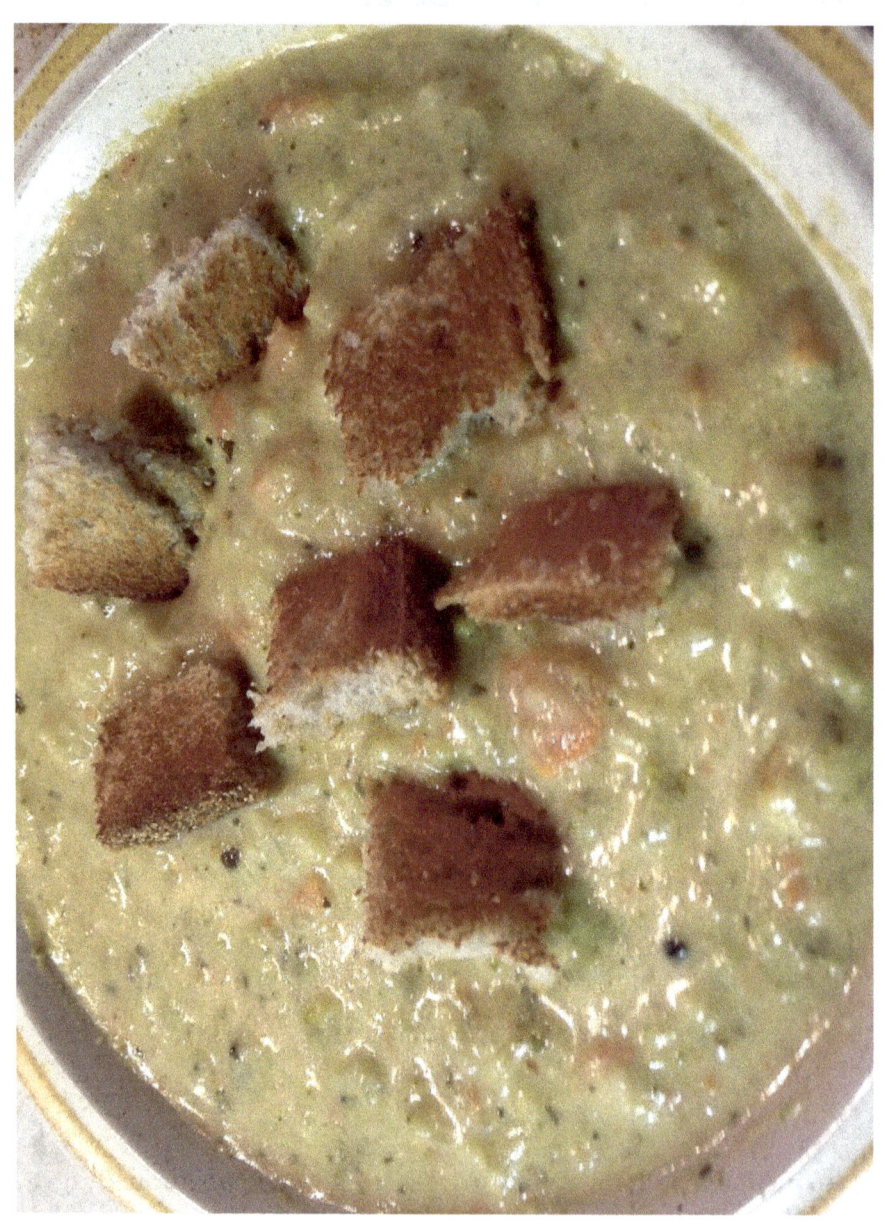

Cilantro And Avocado Platter

Time To Prepare: ten minutes
Time to Cook: 0 minutes
Yield: Servings 6

Ingredients:

- ¼ cup of fresh cilantro, chopped
- ½ a lime, juiced
- 1 big ripe tomato, chopped
- 1 green bell pepper, chopped
- 1 sweet onion, chopped
- 2 avocados, peeled, pitted and diced
- Salt and pepper as required

Directions:

1. Take a moderate-sized container and put in onion, bell pepper, tomato, avocados, lime and cilantro
2. Mix thoroughly and give it a toss
3. Sprinkle with salt and pepper in accordance with your taste
4. Serve and enjoy!

Nutritional Info: ‖ Calories: 126 ‖ Fat: 10g ‖ Carbohydrates: 10g ‖ Protein: 2g

SAUCES AND DRESSINGS

Apple and Tomato Dipping Sauce

Time To Prepare: ten minutes
Time to Cook: 0 minutes
Yield: Servings 2-4

Ingredients:

- ¼ cup of cider vinegar
- ¼ tsp of freshly ground black pepper
- ½ tsp of sea salt
- 1 garlic clove, finely chopped
- 1 large-sized shallot, diced
- 1 tbsp. natural tomato paste
- 1 tbsp. of extra-virgin olive oil
- 1 tbsp. of maple syrup
- 1/8 tsp of ground cloves
- 3 moderate-sized apples, roughly chopped
- 3 moderate-sized tomatoes, roughly chopped

Directions:

1. Put oil into a huge deep cooking pan and heat it up on moderate heat.

2. Put in shallot and cook until light brown for approximately 2 minutes.
3. Stir in the tomato paste, garlic, salt, pepper, and cloves for approximately half a minute. Then put in in the apples, tomatoes, vinegar, and maple syrup.
4. Bring to its boiling point then decrease the heat to allow it to simmer for approximately 30 minutes. Allow to cool for twenty additional minutes before placing the mixture into your blender. Combine the mixture until the desired smoothness is achieved.
5. Keep in a mason jar or an airtight container; place in your fridge for maximum 5 days.
6. Serve it on a burger or with fries.

Nutritional Info: ‖ Calories: 142 kcal ‖ Protein: 3 g ‖ Fat: 3.46 g ‖ Carbohydrates: 26.93 g

Balsamic Vinaigrette

Time To Prepare: ten minutes
Time to Cook: 0 minutes
Yield: Servings 2-4

Ingredients:

- ¼ tsp of freshly ground black pepper
- ½ cup of extra-virgin olive oil
- ½ cup of rice vinegar
- 1 clove of freshly minced garlic
- 1 tbsp. of honey or maple syrup
- 1 tsp of sea or kosher salt
- 2 tsp of Dijon mustard

Directions:

1. Put all ingredients in a mason jar and cover firmly. Shake thoroughly until all ingredients are blended.
2. Keep in your fridge for minimum 30 minutes before you serve to keep its freshness.
3. Serve with a salad or as your meat marinate.

Nutritional Info: ‖ Calories: 147 kcal ‖ Protein: 1.85 g ‖ Fat: 13.21 g ‖ Carbohydrates: 4.02 g

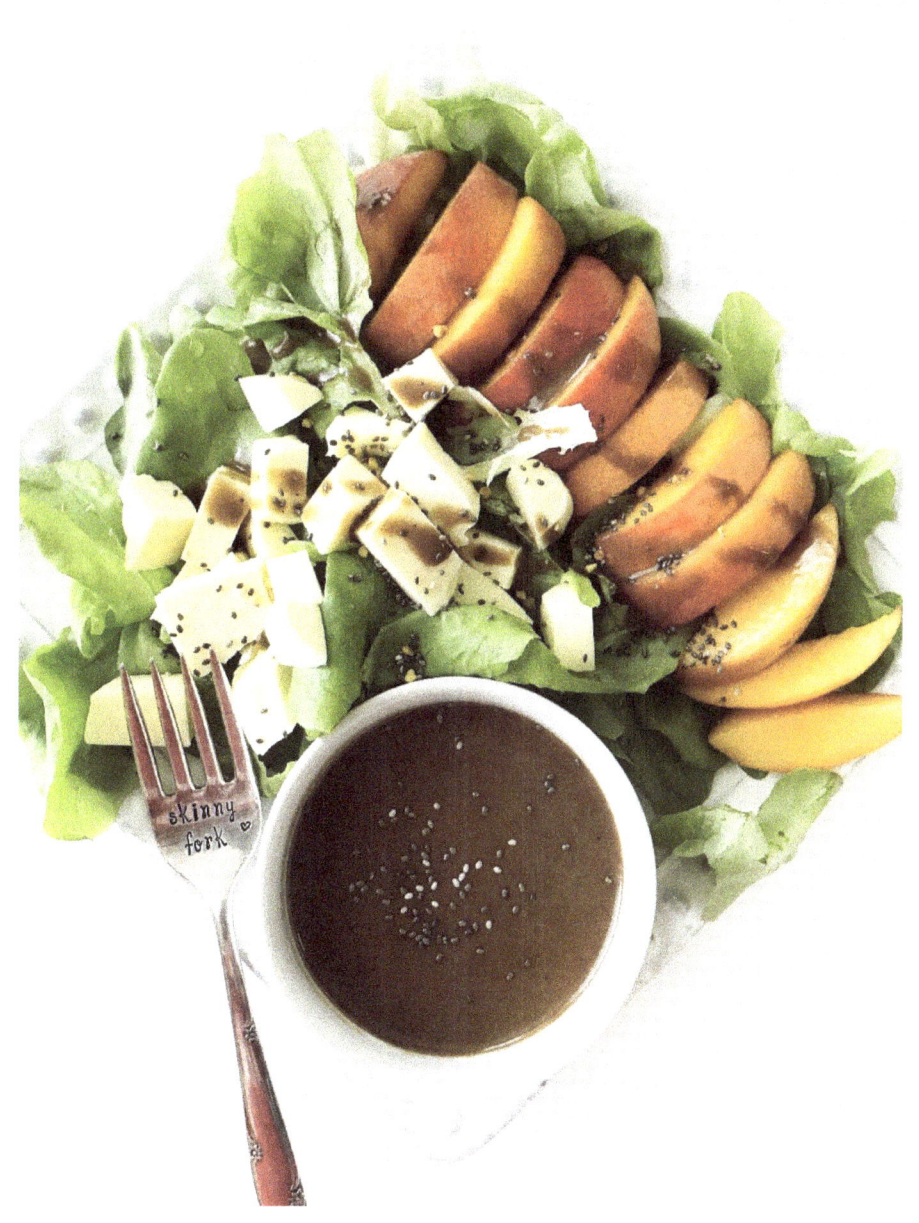

SNACKS

Almond and Honey Homemade Bar

Time To Prepare: fifteen minutes + thirty minutes refrigerator time
Time to Cook: fifteen minutes
Yield: Servings 8

Ingredients:

- ¼ cup almond butter
- ¼ cup honey
- ¼ cup sugar (or another sweetener to your taste in adjusted amount)
- ¼ cup sunflower seeds
- ½ teaspoon vanilla extract
- 1 cup oats
- 1 cup whole-grain puffed cereal (unsweetened)
- 1 tbsp. flaxseeds
- 1 tbsp. sesame seeds
- 1/3 cup apricots (dried and chopped)
- 1/3 cup currants
- 1/3 cup raisins (chopped)
- 1/8 tsp salt

- A ¼ cup of almonds

Directions:

1. Preheat your oven to 350 degrees Fahrenheit.
2. Place a baking paper to an 8-inch pan or coat it with cooking spray/oil.
3. Combine the almonds, oats, and seeds and spread the mixture on a rimmed baking sheet.
4. Bake the mixture until you notice that the oats are mildly toasted (for approximately ten minutes).
5. Move the mixture to a container.
6. Put in cereal, raisins, currants, and apricots to the container.
7. Toss thoroughly to blend.
8. Mix honey, almond butter, vanilla, salt, and sugar in a deep cooking pan.
9. Heat on moderate heat. Stir regularly for 2-5 minutes until you see light bubbles.
10. Once you notice the bubbles, pour the mixture over the dry mixture with apricots and oats you prepared previously.
11. Mix thoroughly using a spatula. There mustn't be any dry spots.
12. Move the new mixture to the previously prepared pan.
13. Push it to the pan to make a firm and flat layer.
14. Place in your refrigerator for half an hour
15. Chop the layer into eight equal bars or squares, to your taste.

16. Consume instantly or place in your refrigerator up to seven days.

Nutritional Info: ‖ Calories: 213 kcal ‖ Protein: 6.92 g ‖ Fat: 9.59 g ‖ Carbohydrates: 32.33 g

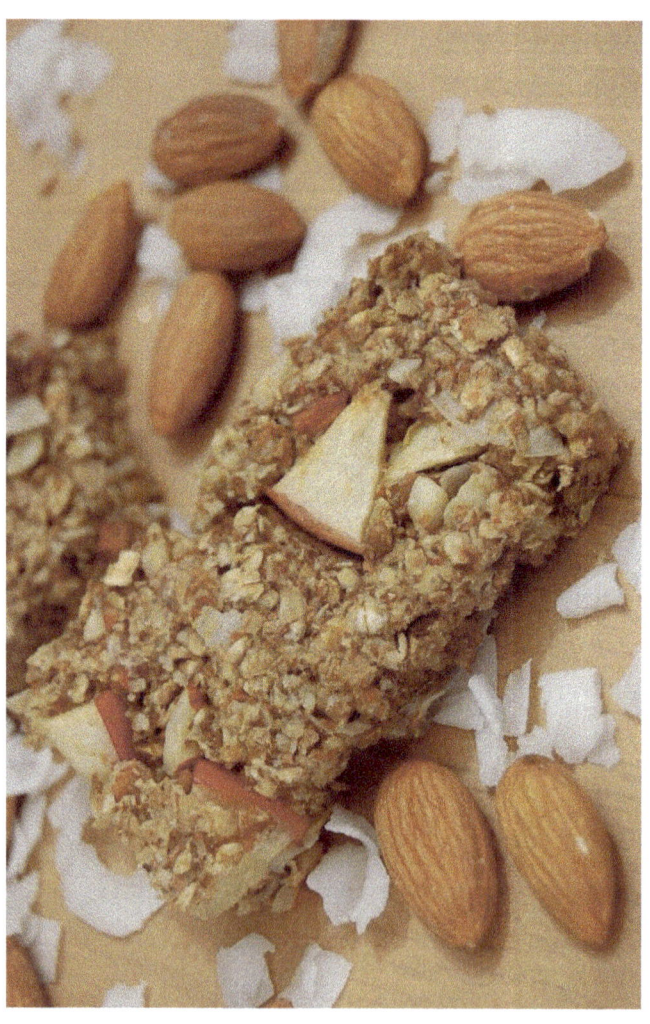

Almonds and Blueberries Yogurt Snack

Time To Prepare: ten minutes
Time to Cook: 0 minutes
Yield: Servings 2

Ingredients:

- 1 ½ cups nonfat Greek yogurt
- 1 cup blueberries
- 20 almonds, chopped

Directions:

1. Take 2 bowls and put in ¾ cup yogurt into each container.
2. Split the blueberries among the bowls and stir.
3. Drizzle half the almonds in each container before you serve.

Nutritional Info: ‖ Calories: 223 kcal ‖ Protein: 6.57 g ‖ Fat: 9.45 g ‖ Carbohydrates: 30.82 g

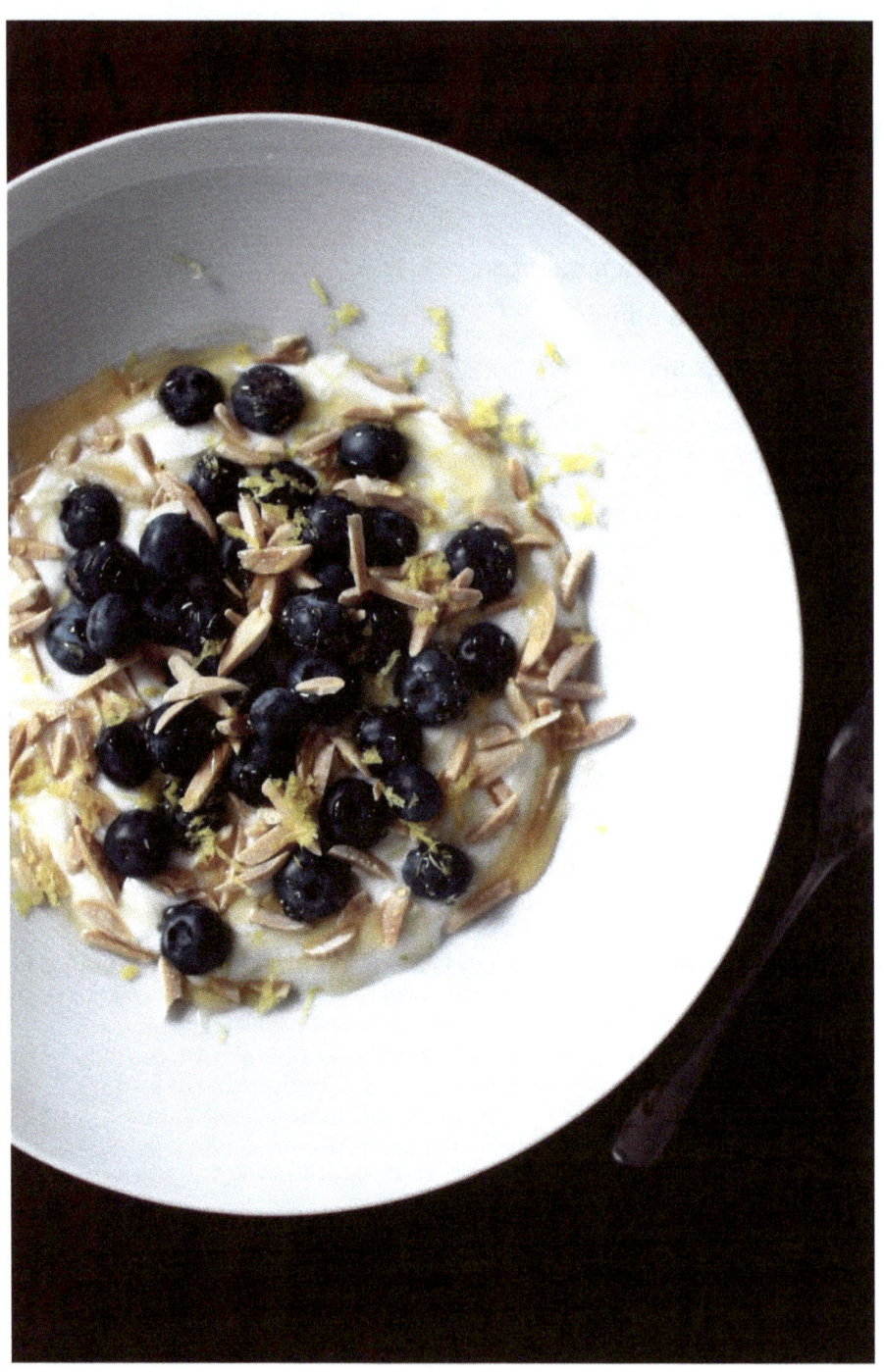

Anti-Inflammatory Key Lime Pie

Time To Prepare: twenty minutes + thirty-five minutes refrigerator time
Time to Cook: 0
Yield: Servings 8

Ingredients:

- ½ cup honey
- ½ cup Medjool dates, chopped and pitted
- 1 cup unsweetened shredded coconut
- 1 cup walnuts
- 1 teaspoon lime zest
- 1/4 teaspoon sea salt
- 3 firm avocados
- 3 tablespoons lime juice
- Lime slices
- Pinch of sea salt

Directions:

1. Use a food processor to put all together the walnuts, coconut, and the salt, then pulse until crudely ground.

2. Place the dates and pulse until the mixture resembles bread crumbs, trying to stick together.
3. Push the mixture into the edges and bottom of a non-stick greased 9-inch pie pan. Use your fingers or the back of a spoon to press the crust into a uniform layer. Bring the crust into the freezer for minimum fifteen minutes while preparing the filling.
4. Use the food processor again and mix the avocado, honey, lime juice, lime zest, and salt. Process until the desired smoothness is achieved.
5. Pour the filling into the now-chilled piecrust and place it in your fridge for about twenty minutes.
6. Decorate using fresh lime slices and serve cold. Store any left overs in your fridge.

Nutritional Info: ‖ Calories: 273 kcal ‖ Protein: 4.19 g ‖ Fat: 18.4 g ‖ Carbohydrates: 28.49 g

Ants on a Log

Time To Prepare: five minutes
Time to Cook: 0 minutes
Yield: Servings 2

Ingredients:

- 3 tablespoons of almond butter
- 3 tablespoons of raisins
- 6 celery sticks

Directions:

1. Spread half a tablespoon of almond butter on each celery stick.
2. Top with half a tablespoon of raisins on each celery stick.
3. Split the celery sticks between two plates, and enjoy!

Nutritional Info: ‖ Total Carbohydrates: 17g ‖ Fiber: 2g ‖ Net Carbohydrates: ‖ Protein: 4g ‖ Total Fat: 14g ‖ Calories: 201

Apple Crisp

Time To Prepare: fifteen minutes
Time to Cook: twenty-five minutes
Yield: Servings 6-8

Ingredients:
Topping:
- 1 ½ cups old-fashioned rolled oats
- 1 teaspoon salt
- ½ cup stevia
- 2 teaspoons ground cinnamon
- 1 cup nuts, crudely chopped
- 3 tablespoon melted coconut oil.
- 1/3 cup almond meal
- 2/3 cup shredded, unsweetened coconut
- 1/4 teaspoon ground nutmeg

Apple filling:
- ½ cup stevia
- 1 tablespoon ground cinnamon
- 1 teaspoon vanilla
- 1/4 cup arrowroot flour
- 1/4 teaspoon salt
- 10 tart apples
- 2 tablespoons fresh-squeezed lemon juice
- 3 tablespoons melted coconut oil

- The zest of 1 orange

Directions:

1. Set the oven to 350 F then grease a 9 by a 13-inch baking pan with coconut oil.
2. Put together the topping ingredients in a container, then mix and save for later.
3. Combine the filling ingredients (except for the apples) in a second big container.
4. Leave the skins on the apples, if you wish. Core them and slice super slim (1/8 inch thick).
5. Toss the apples in the filling ingredients to coat uniformly. Put the apple mixture in a baking pan and spread the topping over it all, pushing down tightly.
6. Put in your oven with a pan underneath to catch any drips.
7. Bake for about twenty-five minutes or until the topping is brown and juices are bubbling. Apples must be tender.
8. Cool slightly on a rack then serve.

Nutritional Info: ‖ Calories: 446 kcal ‖ Protein: 6.15 g ‖ Fat: 27.39 g ‖ Carbohydrates: 57.45 g

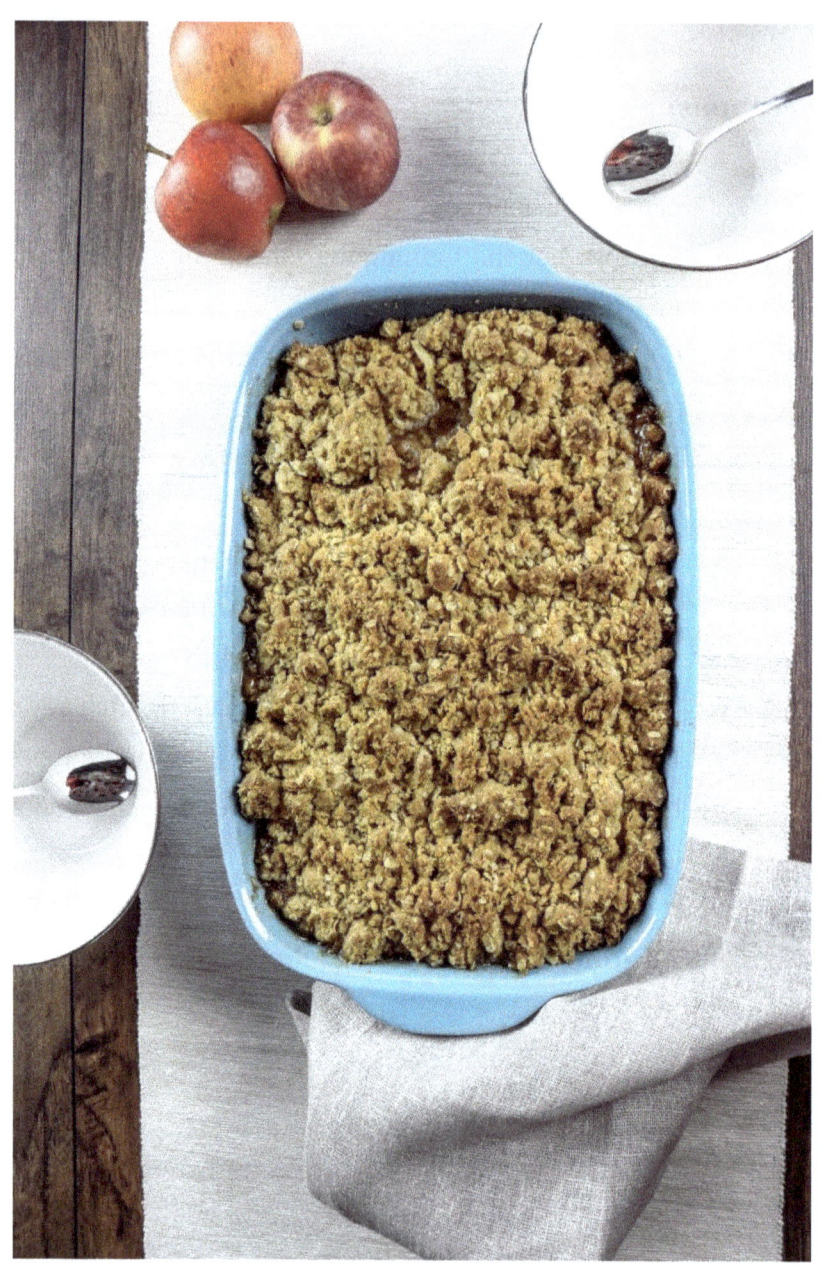

Apple Sauce Treat

Time To Prepare: ten minutes
Time to Cook: 0 minutes
Yield: Servings 1

Ingredients:

- ½ teaspoon cinnamon
- 1 ½ teaspoons toasted slivered almonds
- 1/4 cup low Fat cottage cheese
- 1/4 cup unsweetened applesauce

Directions:

1. Combine the cottage cheese and applesauce in a container, stirring well.
2. Drizzle with cinnamon and mix thoroughly.
3. Drizzle the top with almonds, pick up your spoon, and enjoy.

Nutritional Info: ‖ Calories: 225 kcal ‖ Protein: 16.24 g ‖ Fat: 14.17 g ‖ Carbohydrates: 8.54 g

Avocado and Egg Sandwich

Time To Prepare: ten minutes
Time to Cook: 0 minutes
Yield: Servings 2

Ingredients:

- ½ lime juice
- 1 avocado (ripe)
- 1 egg, organic
- 1 scallion
- 2 radishes
- 2 slices of who wheat, seed bread
- A pinch of salt (sea or Himalayan)
- Black pepper – to your taste
- Mixed seeds – to your choice

Directions:

1. Peel the avocado.
2. Boil the egg (soft boiled).
3. Chop the radishes to thin slices.
4. Dice the scallion (finely).
5. Mix avocado, salt, and lime juice in a container. Mash the mixture meticulously.
6. Spread the mixture onto the bread.
7. Put in some radish.
8. Put tender boiled eggs on top.

9. Put in some scallion, seeds, and pepper.

Nutritional Info: ‖ Calories: 342 kcal ‖ Protein: 12.36 g ‖ Fat: 22.99 g ‖ Carbohydrates: 26.54 g

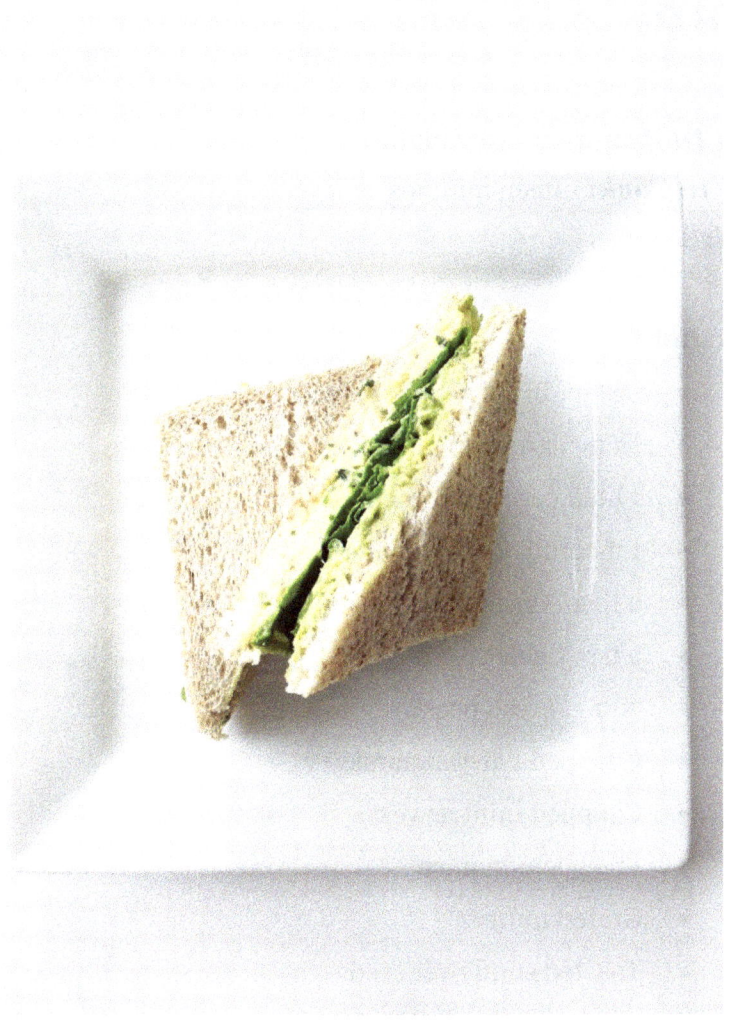

SOUPS AND STEWS

Anti-inflammatory Spring Pea Soup

Time To Prepare: five minutes
Time to Cook: fifteen minutes
Yield: Servings 6

Ingredients:

- ½ tsp. Black pepper powder
- ½ tsp. ground cumin
- 1 liter Vegetable stock
- 1 medium Chopped onion
- 2 tbsp. Coconut oil
- 2 tsp. Celtic sea salt
- 700 g. Fresh peas
- Chopped flat-leaf parsley
- Chopped mint leaves
- Fresh lemon juice
- Grated nutmeg
- Toasted sunflower seeds

Directions:

1. Warm the coconut oil in a pan set on moderate heat.

2. Mix in onions and stir fry for approximately five minutes.
3. Put in the stock and raise the heat. Throw in fresh peas and cook for five minutes. If you're using frozen peas, it should take half the time.
4. Pour in the lemon juice, salt, pepper, herbs, and spices. Stirring continuously
5. Remove the heat and allow it to cool before running it through a food processor to whatever consistency you prefer.
6. Serve with sunflower seed sprinkles and mint or parsley leaves.
7. Enjoy!

Nutritional Info: Calories: 115 kcal ‖ Protein: 5 g ‖ Fat: 5.91 g ‖ Carbohydrates: 11.8 g

Anti-Inflammatory Sweet Potato Soup

Time To Prepare: twenty minutes
Time to Cook: thirty minutes
Yield: Servings 8

Ingredients:

- 1 13.66-ounce can lite coconut milk
- 1 big zucchini, cut width-wise
- 1 garlic clove
- 1 liter low-sodium vegetable stock
- 1 tablespoon sweet yellow curry powder
- 1 teaspoon black pepper
- 1 teaspoon cayenne pepper
- 1 teaspoon turmeric
- 1 white onion
- 2 moderate-sized white potatoes,
- 3 moderate-sized sweet potatoes,
- 3/4 tablespoons salt
- 4 cups of hot water
- 4 tablespoons olive oil
- A pinch of cinnamon
- A pinch of cloves
-

Directions:

1. Prepare every one of your vegetables by cutting, cleaning & cubing. Put in a safe spot.
2. To a large pot, include 4 tablespoons of additional virgin olive oil. Allow it to heat up swiftly; at that point, include your white onion. Allow it to sweat for minimum five minutes on low warmth.
3. Put in all your flavoring & garlic. Give it a decent mix; at that point, including the potatoes.
4. Allow these cook on moderate heat for around five minutes to get a pleasant darker shading. Continue blending to abstain from consuming.
5. Put in your stalk & water, warm it to the point of boiling & then stew for around 20-twenty-five minutes. Part of the way through the stewing procedure, include your zucchini.
6. After 20-twenty-five minutes, include your coconut milk. Before pouring the soup to the blender, do a fork content to guarantee your potatoes are cooked.
7. Use your blender to purée the soup. Embellishment with lemon juice, dark pepper & herbs & flavors of your preference.

Nutritional Info: Calories: 281 kcal ‖ Protein: 4.1 g ‖ Fat: 20.22 g ‖ Carbohydrates: 23.8 g

Bacon & Cheese Soup

Time To Prepare: fifteen minutes
Time to Cook: forty minutes
Yield: Servings 6

Ingredients:

- ½ cup sour cream, for serving
- ½ teaspoon cumin
- ½ teaspoon onion powder
- ½ teaspoon paprika
- 1 cup heavy cream
- 1 cup shredded cheddar cheese
- 1 pound of lean ground beef
- 1 tablespoon coconut oil, for cooking
- 1 teaspoon garlic powder
- 1 yellow onion, chopped
- 6 cups beef broth
- 6 slices uncured bacon

Directions:

1. Put in the coconut oil to a frying pan and cook the bacon until crunchy. Allow the bacon to cool and cut into little pieces. Set aside.
2. Once cooked, put in the lean ground beef to the same frying pan with the bacon fat and cook until browned.

3. Put in the onions and cook for an extra two to three minutes.
4. Put in all the ingredients minus the bacon, heavy cream, sour cream and cheese to a stockpot and stir. Cook for about twenty-five minutes.
5. Warm the heavy cream, and then put in the warmed cream and cheese and serve with the bacon and a spoonful of sour cream.

Nutritional Info: Calories: 498 ‖ Carbohydrates: 5g ‖ Fiber: 1g Net ‖ Carbohydrates: 4g ‖ Fat: 34g ‖ Protein: 41g

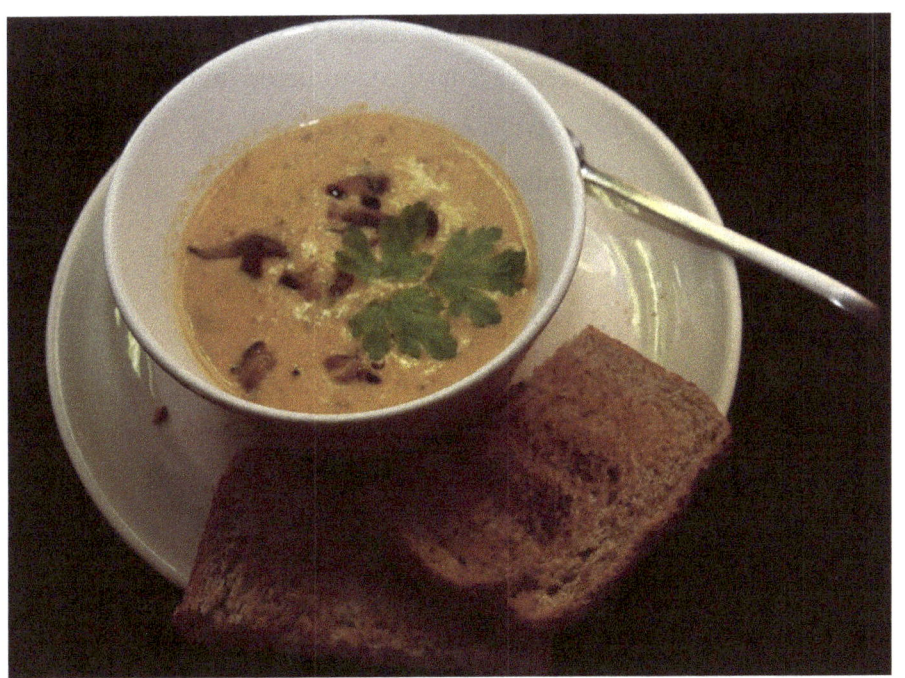

Beef And Veggie Soup

Time To Prepare: ten minutes
Time to Cook: twenty minutes
Yield: Servings 8

Ingredients:

- ½ cup heavy whipping cream
- ½ cup onion, chopped
- 1 (8 ounces / 227 g) package cream cheese, softened
- 1 pound (454 g) ground beef
- 1 tablespoon ground cumin
- 1 teaspoon chili powder
- 2 (10 ounces / 284 g) cans diced tomatoes and green chiles
- 2 (14.5 ounces / 411 g) cans beef broth
- 2 cloves garlic, minced
- 2 teaspoons salt, or to taste

Directions:

1. Position the ground beef, chopped onion, and garlic in a pot, stir until blended well. Cook on moderate to high heat for five to seven minutes or until the beef is thoroughly browned. Stir continuously.
2. Discard the grease extract from the beef, then put in chili powder and cumin, and cook for an extra two minutes. Stir continuously.

3. Put in the cream cheese to the pot and cook for three to five minutes more, then fold in the tomatoes and green chiles, beef broth, heavy whipping cream, and salt, and cook for about ten minutes to cook through. Keep stirring during the cooking.
4. Serve the soup in a big serving container. Allow to stand for a couple of minutes before you serve.

Nutritional Info: calories: 288 ‖ total fat: 24g ‖ carbs: 5.4g ‖ protein: 13.4g ‖ Cholesterol: 85mg ‖ Sodium: 1310mg

Broccoli Cheddar & Bacon Soup

Time To Prepare: ten minutes
Time to Cook: ten minutes
Yield: Servings 6

Ingredients:

- ¼ teaspoon black pepper
- ½ teaspoon salt
- ½ white onion, chopped
- 1 cup broccoli florets finely chopped
- 1 cup heavy cream
- 1 cup shredded cheddar cheese
- 2 cloves garlic, chopped
- 2 cups chicken broth
- 3 slices cooked bacon, crumbled for serving

Directions:

1. Put in all the ingredients minus the heavy cream, cheddar cheese and bacon to a stockpot on moderate heat.
2. Heat to a simmer and cook for 5 minutes.
3. Warm the cream, and then put in the warm cream and cheddar cheese. Whisk until the desired smoothness is achieved.
4. Serve with crumbled bacon.

Nutritional Info: Calories: 220 ‖ Carbohydrates: 4g ‖ Fiber: 1g Net ‖ Carbohydrates: 3g ‖ Fat: 18g ‖ Protein: 11g

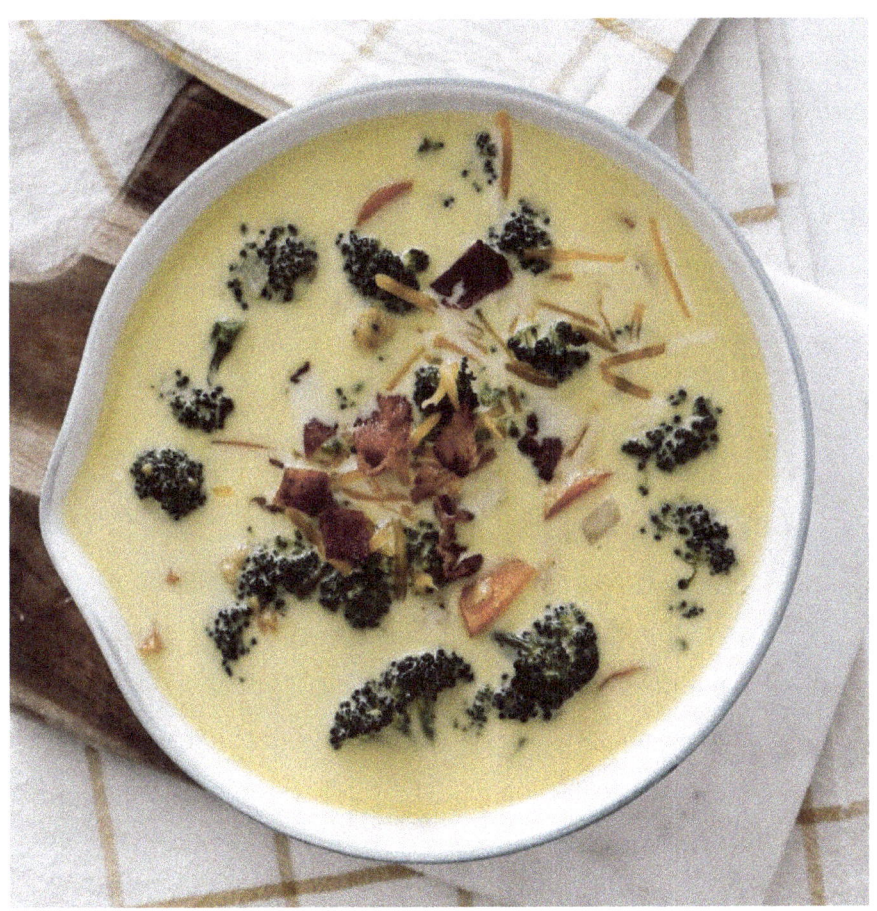

Broccoli Soup with Gorgonzola Cheese

Time To Prepare: ten minutes
Time to Cook: thirty minutes
Yield: Servings 4

Ingredients:

- ½ cup 18% cream
- 1 big broccoli, divided into little roses
- 1 flat teaspoon of sweet pepper
- 1 onion, diced
- 1 tablespoon of chopped fresh basil
- 1 tablespoon of chopped parsley
- 1 tablespoon of oil
- 150 g Gorgonzola cheese, diced
- 2 potatoes, peeled and diced
- 4 tablespoons of almond flakes roasted in a dry pan
- 5 garlic cloves, chopped
- 750 ml broth
- a pinch of sugar
- pumpkin oil (not necessary)
- salt and pepper

Directions:
1. In a big deep cooking pan, warm the oil on moderate heat, put the onion and garlic, and fry it until the vitrified glass onion.
2. Then put the broccoli with potatoes, pour the broth and cook for approximately fifteen-twenty minutes until the vegetables become tender. Put in basil, parsley, sugar, pepper, and pepper to taste.
3. Put in cheese and cream, and when the cheese dissolves, blend with a blender until the desired smoothness is achieved. Sprinkle with salt and pepper if required.
4. Serve the soup sprinkled with almond flakes and sprinkled with pumpkin oil.

Nutritional Info: Calories: 382 kcal ‖ Protein: 13.06 g ‖ Fat: 18.93 g ‖ Carbohydrates: 41.65 g

Brown Rice and Shitake Miso Soup with Scallion

Time To Prepare: ten minutes
Time to Cook: forty-five minutes
Yield: Servings 4

Ingredients:

- ½ teaspoon salt
- 1 (1½-inch) piece fresh ginger, peeled and cut
- 1 cup medium-grain brown rice
- 1 cup thinly cut shiitake mushroom caps
- 1 garlic clove, minced
- 1 tablespoon white miso
- 2 scallions, thinly cut
- 2 tablespoons finely chopped fresh cilantro
- 2 tablespoons sesame oil

Directions:

1. In a large pot, heat the oil on moderate to high heat.
2. Put in the mushrooms, garlic, and ginger and sauté until the mushrooms start to tenderize, approximately five minutes.
3. Place the rice and stir to uniformly coat with the oil.
4. Put in 2 cups of water and salt and place it to its boiling point.

5. Reduce the heat then cook until the rice is soft, thirty to forty minutes.
6. Use a little of the soup broth to tenderize the miso, then mix it into the pot until well mixed.
7. Stir in the scallions and cilantro, then serve.

Nutritional Info: Calories: 265 ‖ Total Fat: 8g ‖ Total Carbohydrates: 43g ‖ Sugar: 2g ‖ Fiber: 3g ‖ Protein: 5g ‖ Sodium: 456mg

Buffalo Sauce And Turkey Soup

Time To Prepare: five minutes
Time to Cook: ten minutes
Yield: Servings 4

Ingredients:
- ⅓ cup buffalo sauce
- 2 cups turkey, cooked, shredded
- 3 tablespoons butter, melted
- 4 cups chicken broth
- 4 ounces (113 g) cream cheese
- 4 tablespoons cilantro, chopped
- From The Cupboard:
- Salt and freshly ground black pepper, to taste

Directions:
1. Place the buffalo sauce, cream cheese, and melted butter in a blender, and process until the desired smoothness is achieved.
2. Pour the buffalo sauce mixture in a deep cooking pan, and put in the chicken broth. Heat the soup using high heat until hot and nearly boil off but not boil. Keep stirring during the heating.
3. Put in the shredded turkey, and drizzle with salt and black pepper. Cook for five minutes or until the desired smoothness is achieved. Stir continuously.

4. Ladle the soup into a big container and top with chopped cilantro before you serve.

Nutritional Info: calories: 409 ‖ total fat: 29.7g ‖ net carbs: 9.2g ‖ protein: 26.4g

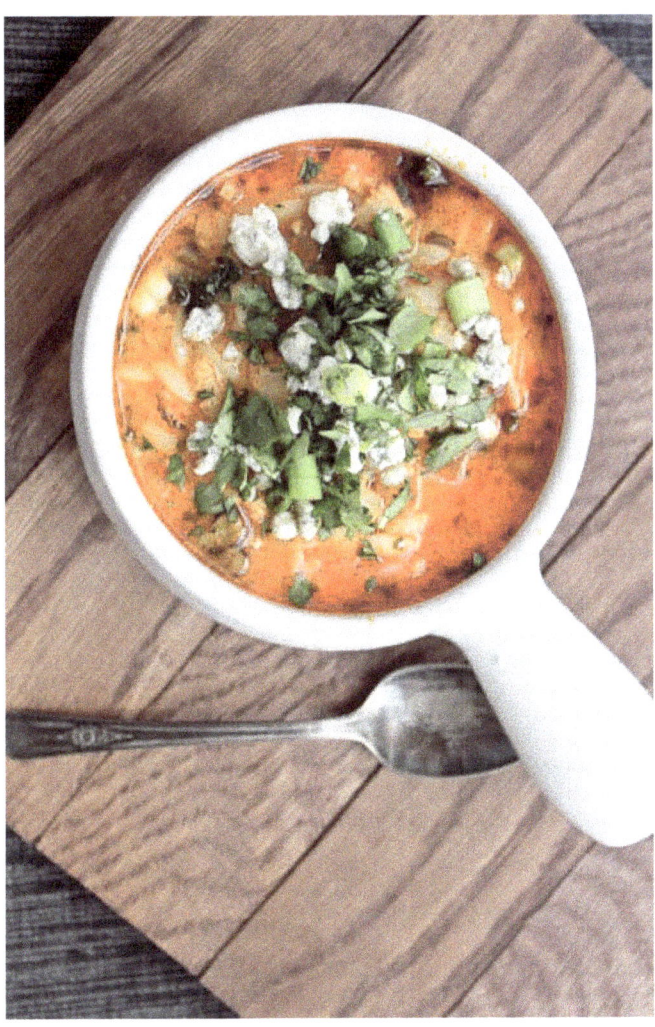

Butternut Squash Soup with Shrimp

Time To Prepare: ten minutes
Time to Cook: twenty minutes
Yield: Servings 4

Ingredients:

- ¼ cup slivered almonds (not necessary)
- ¼ teaspoon freshly ground black pepper
- 1 cup unsweetened almond milk
- 1 garlic clove, cut
- 1 pound cooked peeled shrimp, thawed if required
- 1 small red onion, finely chopped
- 1 teaspoon salt
- 1 teaspoon turmeric
- 2 cups peeled butternut squash cut into ¼-inch dice
- 2 tablespoons finely chopped fresh flat-leaf parsley
- 2 teaspoons grated or minced lemon zest
- 3 cups vegetable broth
- 3 tablespoons unsalted butter

Directions:

1. In a large pot, melt the butter on high heat.

2. Put in the onion, garlic, turmeric, salt, and pepper and sauté until the vegetables are tender and translucent, five to seven minutes.
3. Put in the broth and squash and bring to its boiling point.
4. Reduce the heat and cook until the squash has tenderized, approximately five minutes.
5. Put in the shrimp and almond milk and cook until thoroughly heated, approximately 2 minutes.
6. Drizzle with the almonds (if using), parsley, and lemon zest before you serve.

Nutritional Info: Calories: 275 ‖ Total Fat: 12g ‖ Total Carbohydrates: 12g ‖ Sugar: 3g ‖ Fiber: 2g; ‖ Protein: 30g ‖ Sodium: 1665mg

Cannellini Bean Soup

Time To Prepare: twenty-five minutes
Time to Cook: thirty minutes
Yield: Servings 6

Ingredients:
- 1 bunch red Swiss chard
- 1 cannellini beans
- 1 clove garlic (minced)
- 1 onion (chopped)
- 1 tablespoon extra-virgin olive oil
- 1/4 teaspoon nutmeg (grated)
- 1/8 teaspoon red pepper flakes (crushed)
- 2 ounces Parmesan cheese rind
- 2 slices smoked bacon (chopped)
- 2 tablespoons chopped sun-dried tomatoes
- 5 big sage leaves (minced)
- 5 leaves basil (chopped)
- 6 cups chicken broth

Directions:
1. Cook the bacon with garlic, onion, nutmeg, and red pepper flakes for five minutes.
2. Pour in beans, chicken broth, sun-dried tomatoes, and Parmesan cheese rind, simmering for about ten minutes.

3. Put in the cut chard and chard leaves into the soup.
4. Simmer and then put in into bowls with a sprinkle of oil and Parmesan cheese.

Nutritional Info: Calories: 215 kcal ‖ Carbohydrates: 23 g ‖ Fat: 10 g ‖ Protein: 9.7 g

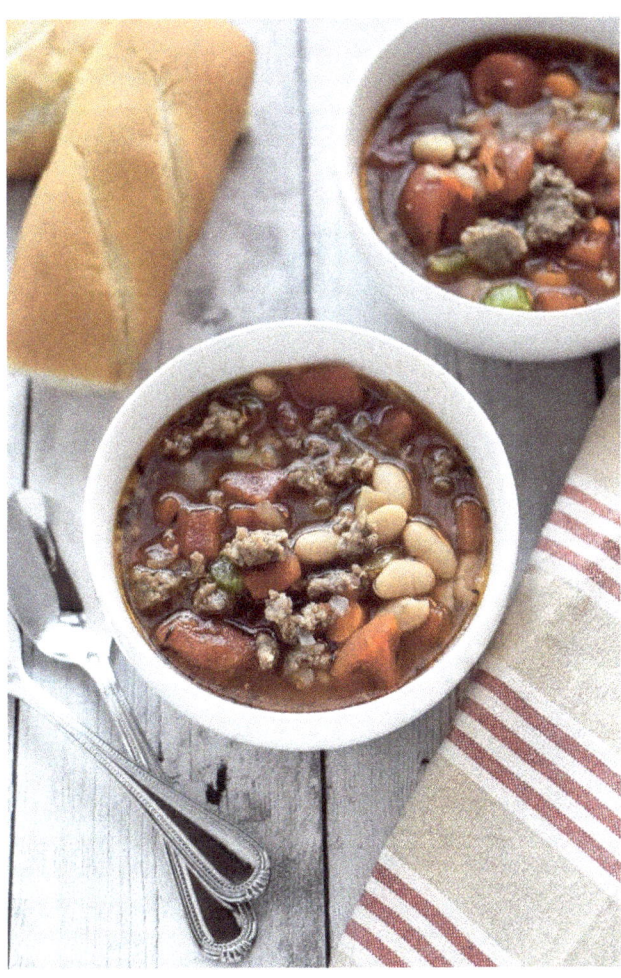

Desserts

Almond Butter Balls Vegan

Time To Prepare: 10 Minutes
Time to Cook: 0 0 Minute
Yield: Servings 4

Ingredients:

- 12 dates, pitted and diced
- 2 and a ½ tablespoon of almond butter
- 1/3 cup of unsweetened shredded coconut

Directions:

1. Take a container and put in dates, almond butter, and coconut. Mix thoroughly
2. Use the mixture to make small balls
3. Store them in the refrigerator and chill them
4. Enjoy!

Nutritional Info: ‖ Calories: 62 Cal ‖ Fat: 3 g ‖ Carbohydrates:8 g ‖ Protein:1 g

Almond Cookies

Time To Prepare: fifteen min
Time to Cook: fifteen min
Yield: Servings 12

Ingredients:

- ½ tsp honey
- ½ tsp vanilla
- 1.7oz / 50g coconut butter
- 14oz / 400g non-wheat flour
- 1tsp baking powder
- 1tsp baking soda
- 3.5oz / 100g tahini
- Salt

Directions:

1. Combine the flour, soda, salt, baking powder together.
2. Mix tahini and coconut butter together and put in 2 tbsp. water in the same container.
3. Put in honey, vanilla to the tahini mixture and blend it well with a mixer.
4. Preheat the oven (180C/356F) and place a baking sheet on it.
5. Put in 24 tablespoons of the mixture onto the baking sheet and allow it to bake in your oven for 11-fifteen minutes.
6. Allow it to get cold a little bit before you serve.

Nutritional Info: ‖ Calories: 112 ‖ Carbohydrates:18 g ‖ Protein: 3.2 g ‖ Fat: 1.6 g ‖ Sugar: 23.1 g ‖ Fiber: 7.4 g ‖ Sodium: 28 mg

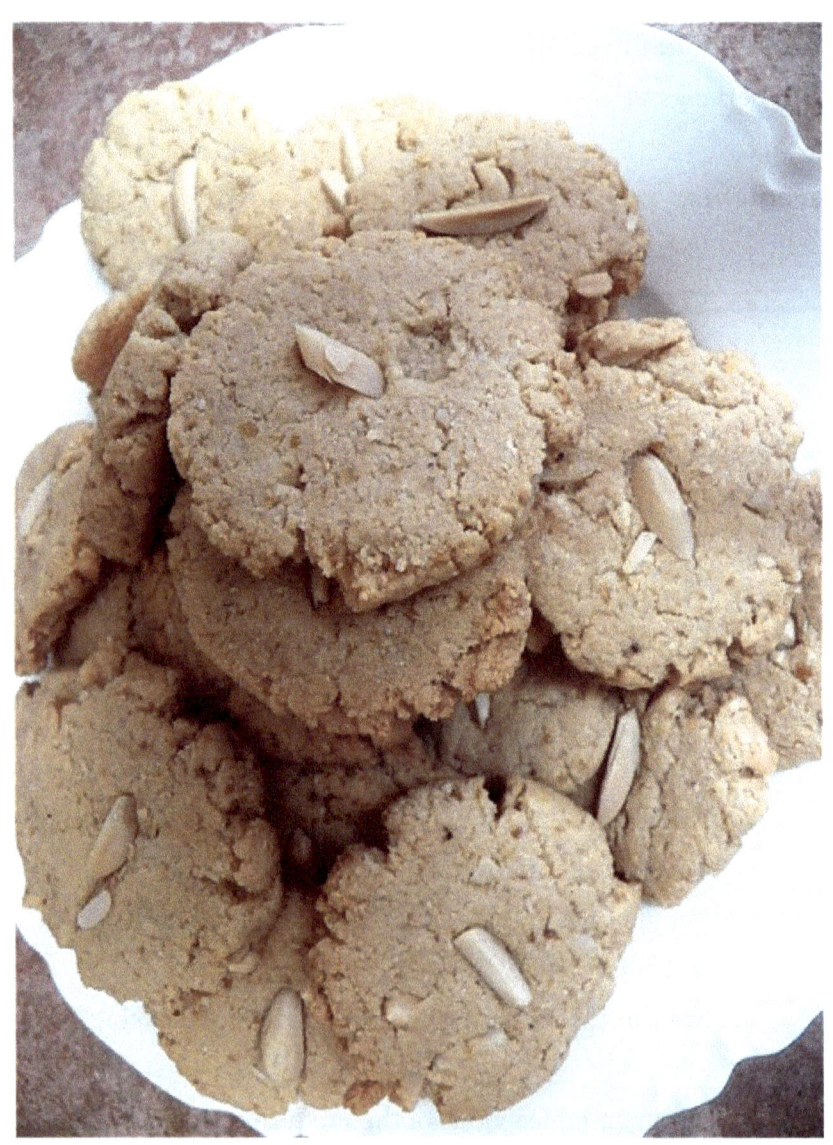

Anti-Inflammatory Apricot Squares

Time To Prepare: twenty minutes
Time to Cook: 0 minute
Yield: Servings 8

Ingredients:

- 1 cup apricot, chopped
- 1 cup apricot, dried
- 1 cup macadamia nuts, chopped
- 1 cup shredded coconut, dried
- 1 teaspoon vanilla extract
- 1/3 cup turmeric powder

Directions:

1. Put all ingredients in a food processor
2. Pulse until the desired smoothness is achieved
3. Put the mixture into a square pan and press uniformly

Best enjoyed chilled.

Nutritional Info: ‖ Calories: 201 ‖ Fat: 15g ‖ Carbohydrates: 17g ‖ Protein: 3g

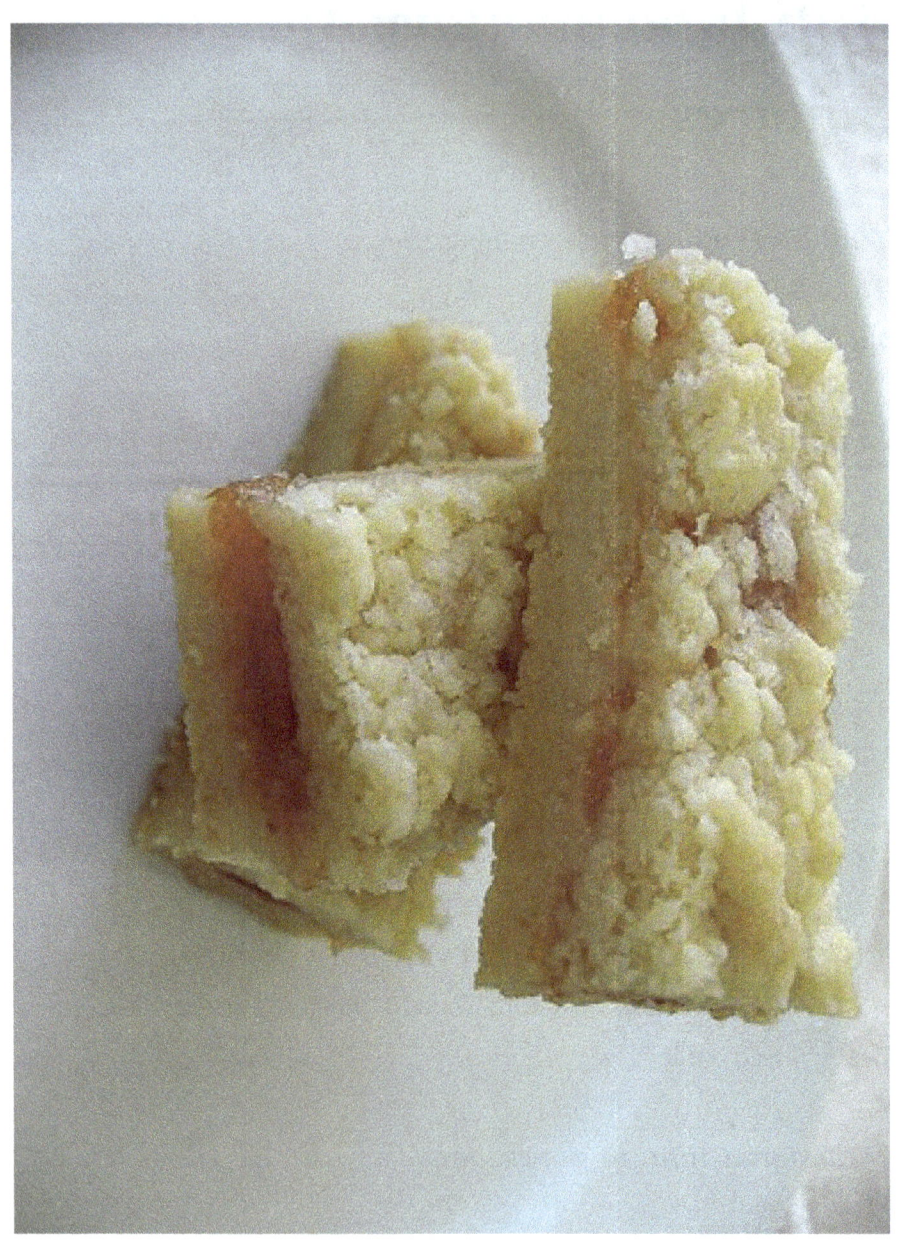

Apple Fritters

Time To Prepare: fifteen minutes
Time to Cook: ten minutes
Yield: Servings 4

Ingredients:

- ½ cup cashew milk
- 1 apple, cored, peeled, and chopped
- 1 cup all-purpose flour
- 1 egg
- 1½ teaspoons of baking powder
- 2 tablespoons of stevia sugar

Directions:

1. Preheat the air fryer to 175 degrees C or 350 degrees F.
2. Place parchment paper at the bottom of your fryer. Line with cooking spray.
3. Mix together ¼ cup sugar, flour, baking powder, egg, milk, and salt in a container.
4. Mix well by stirring.
5. Drizzle 2 tablespoons of sugar on the apples. Coat well.
6. Mix the apples into your flour mixture.
7. Use a cookie scoop and drop the fritters with it to the air fryer basket's bottom.
8. Now air fry for five minutes.

9. Flip the fritters once and fry for another three minutes. They must be golden.

Nutritional Info: Calories 307 ‖ Carbohydrates: 65g ‖ Cholesterol: 48mg ‖ Total Fat: 3g ‖ Protein: 5g ‖ Sugar: 39g ‖ Fiber: 2g ‖ Sodium: 248mg

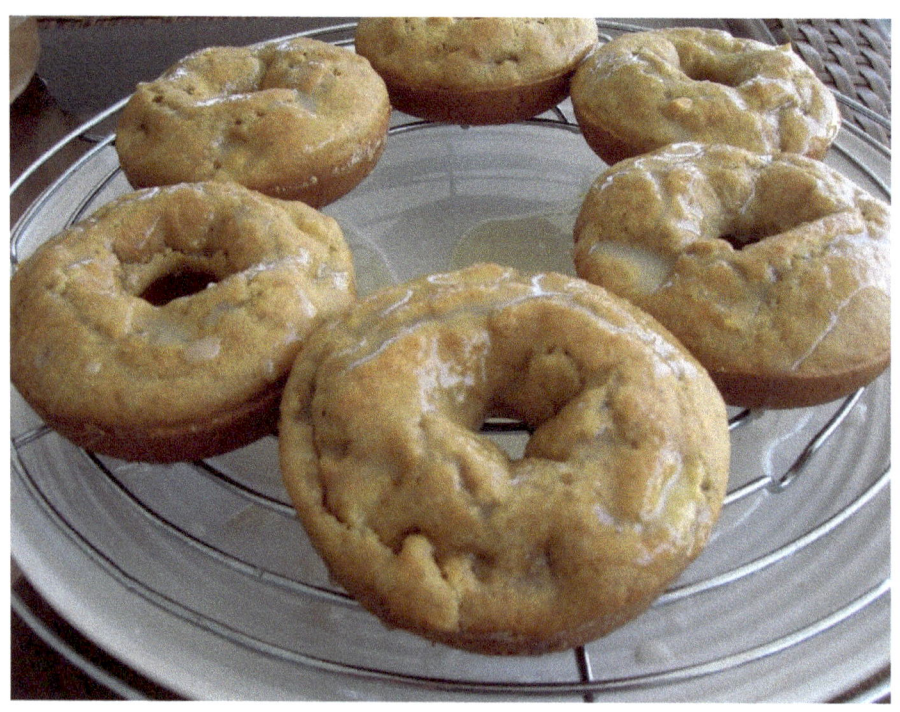

Avocado Brownies

Time To Prepare: 10 Minutes
Time to Cook: 25 Minutes
Yield: Servings 16

Ingredients:

- ¼ tsp. Sea Salt
- ½ cup Applesauce, unsweetened
- ½ cup Cocoa Powder, Dutch-processed & unsweetened
- ½ cup Coconut Flour
- ½ cup Maple Syrup
- 1 Avocado, big
- 1 tap. Vanilla Extract
- 1 tsp. Baking Soda
- 3 Eggs, large

Directions:

1. First, preheat your oven to 350 ° F.
2. Next, place avocado, vanilla, applesauce, and maple syrup in a high-speed blender and blend for a couple of minutes or until the desired smoothness is achieved.
3. After this, move the smooth mixture to a big mixing container.
4. To this, mix in the eggs and mix until whisked well.
5. Next, spoon in the coconut flour, sea salt, and cocoa powder to the mixture.

6. Give a good stir until everything comes together.
7. Now, pour the mixture to a greased baking dish and bake for 23 to twenty-five minutes or until cooked.
8. Finally, take off from the oven and let it cool for fifteen to twenty minutes before you serve.

Nutritional Info: ‖ Calories: 91Kcal ‖ Protein: 1.9g ‖ Carbohydrates: 12.1g ‖ Fat: 4.3g

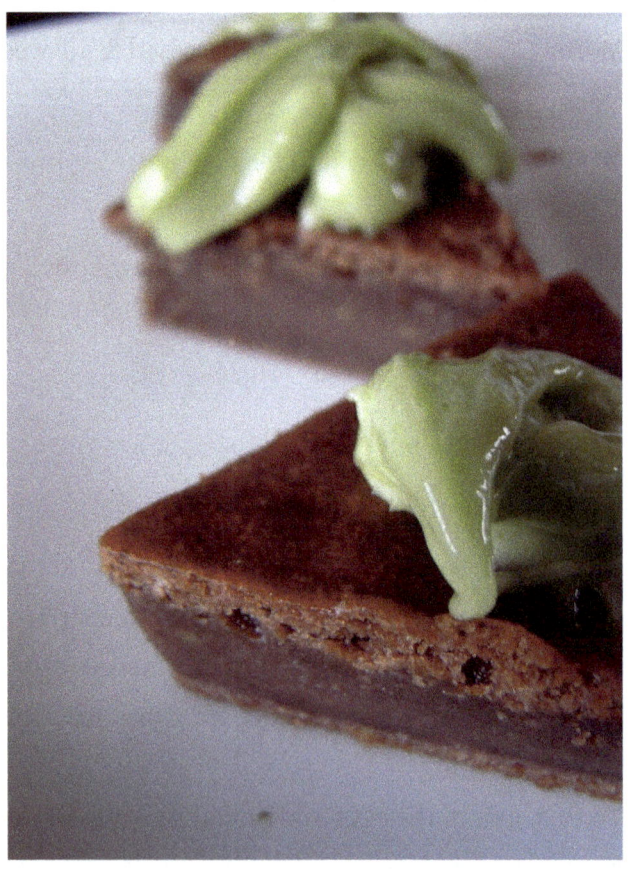

Avocado Chia Parfait

Time To Prepare: five minutes
Time to Cook: twenty minutes
Yield: Servings 2

Ingredients:

- ⅛ teaspoon nutmeg powder
- ½ teaspoon cinnamon powder
- ¾ teaspoon cinnamon powder
- 1 banana, mashed
- 1 tablespoon cashew nuts, chopped
- 1¼ cups almond milk
- 2 avocados, diced
- 2 tablespoons chia seeds
- 2 tablespoons pumpkin seeds
- For the Avocado Jam
- For the Parfait Base
- Pinch of sea salt

Directions:

1. In a container, mix almond milk, banana, nutmeg powder, cinnamon powder, and pumpkin seeds. Mix until well blended. Chill in your refrigerator.
2. In the meantime, put the deep cooking pan on moderate heat. Mix avocados, nutmeg powder, cinnamon powder,

and salt. Bring to its boiling point. Allow simmering for about twenty minutes.
3. Remove the heat. Mash half of the jam using a wooden spoon. Allow to cool. Set aside.
4. Ladle 2 tablespoons of parfait base and apple jam into parfait glasses. Decorate using cashew nuts and serve.

Nutritional Info: ∥ Calories: 671 kcal ∥ Protein: 13.13 g ∥ Fat: 54.86 g ∥ Carbohydrates: 43.76 g

Avocado Choco Cake

Time To Prepare: ten minutes
Time to Cook: twenty-five minutes
Yield: Servings 8

Ingredients:

- ¼-tsp sea salt
- ½-cup applesauce, unsweetened
- ½-cup cocoa powder, unsweetened and Dutch-processed
- ½-cup coconut flour
- ½-cup maple syrup
- 1-pc big avocado
- 1-tsp baking soda
- 1-tsp vanilla extract
- 3-pcs big eggs

Directions:

1. Preheat the oven to 350°F. Grease a baking pan with coconut oil.
2. Mix the avocado, vanilla, syrup, and applesauce in a food processor. Blend until meticulously blended.
3. Move the mixture to a big mixing container. Whisk in the eggs. Put in the baking soda, cocoa powder, coconut flour, and sea salt. Mix thoroughly until meticulously blended.
4. Put in the batter in the baking pan. Place the pan in your oven. Bake for about twenty-five minutes.

5. Allow cooling for about twenty minutes before cutting the cake into 16 squares.

Nutritional Info: ‖ Calories: 253 ‖ Fat: 8.4g ‖ Protein: 12.6g ‖ Sodium: 245mg ‖ Total Carbohydrates: 43.9g ‖ Fiber: 12.3g ‖ Net Carbohydrates: 31.6g

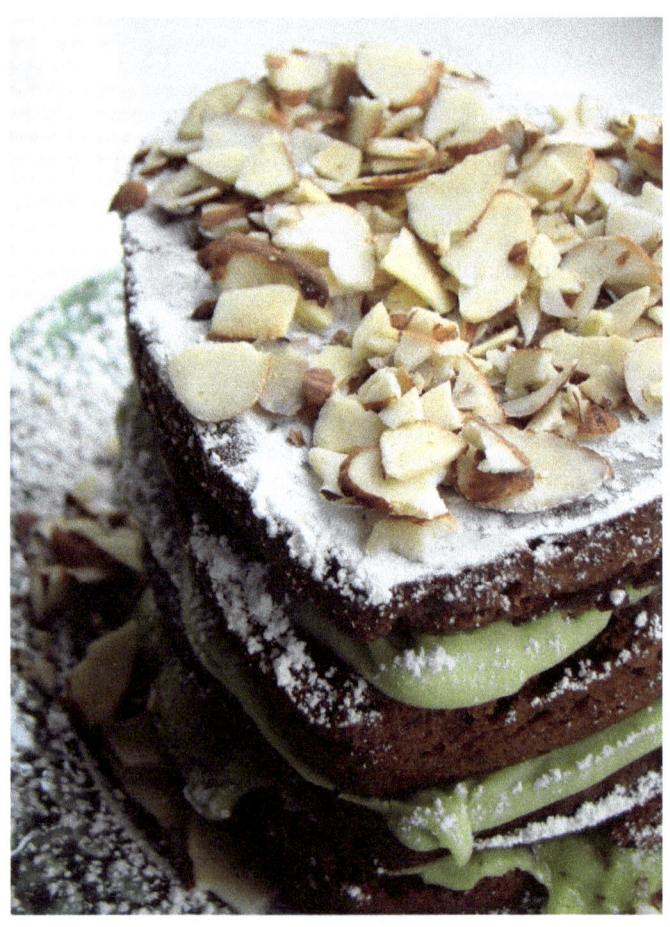

Avocado Chocolate Mousse

Time To Prepare: ten minutes
Time to Cook: 0 minute
Yield: Servings 9

Ingredients:

- ¼ cup espresso beans, ground
- ¼ cup of cocoa powder
- ½ teaspoon salt
- 1 bar dark chocolate
- 1 teaspoon vanilla extract
- 1/8 cup almond milk, unsweetened
- 2 tablespoons raw honey
- 3 ripe avocado, pitted and flesh scooped out
- 6 ounces plain Greek yogurt

Directions:

1. Put all ingredients in a food processor
2. Pulse until the desired smoothness is achieved

Best enjoyed chilled.

Nutritional Info: ‖ Calories: 208 ‖ Fat: 4g ‖ Carbohydrates: 17g ‖ Protein: 5g

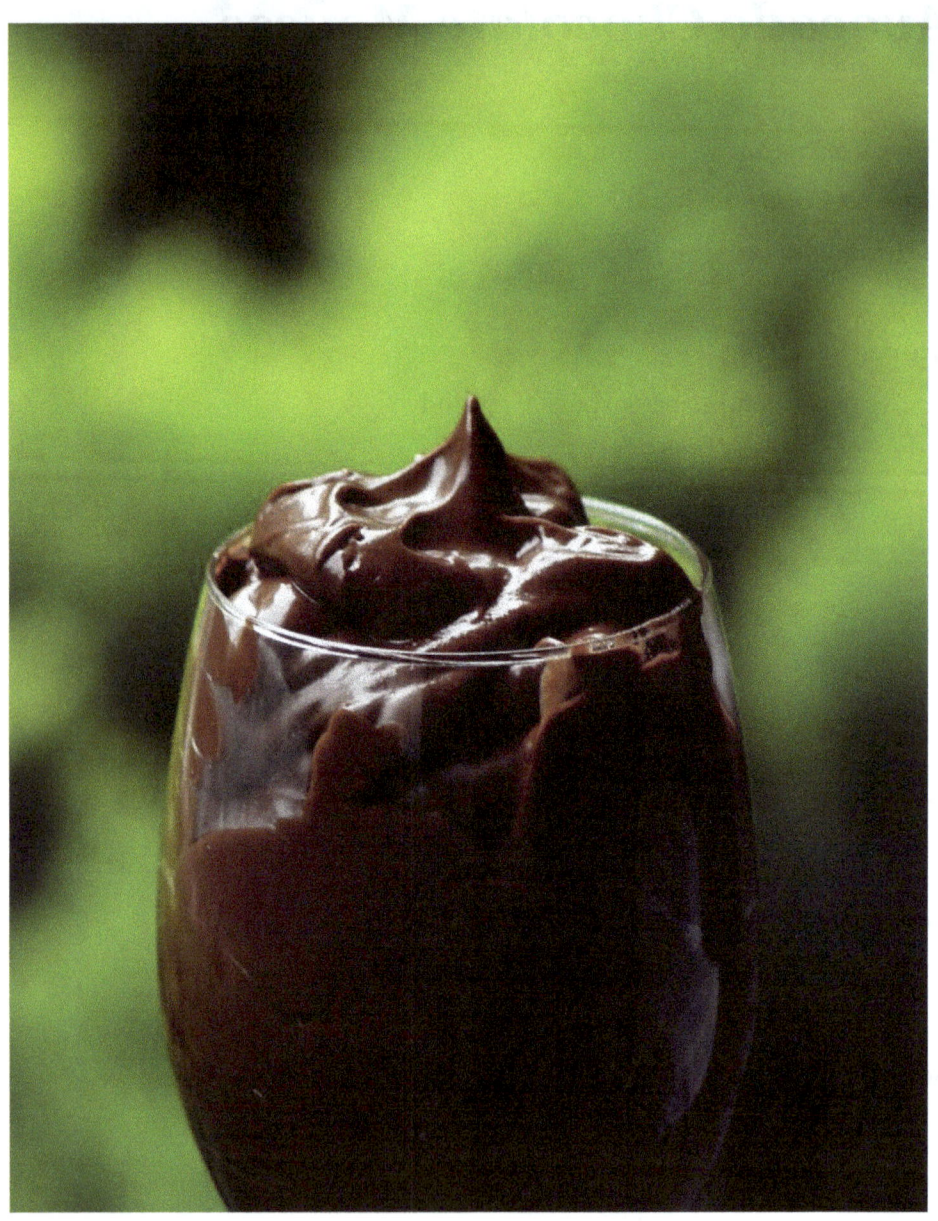

Banana & Avocado Mousse

Time To Prepare: ten minutes
Time to Cook: 0 minutes
Yield: Servings 4

Ingredients:

- ½ cup of fresh lemon juice
- ½ cup of fresh lime juice
- 1 teaspoon of fresh lemon zest, grated finely
- 1 teaspoon of fresh lime zest, grated finely
- 1/3 cup of raw honey
- 2 cups of bananas (peeled and chopped)
- 2 ripe avocados (peeled, pitted, and chopped)

Directions:

1. Combine all ingredients in a blender and pulse to puree.
2. Move the mousse to four serving glasses.
3. Place in your fridge for around three hours before eating.

Nutritional Info: ‖ Calories: 368 ‖ Fat: 20.1g ‖ Carbohydrates: 50.2g ‖ Sugar: 33.6g ‖ Protein: 3.1g ‖ Sodium: 14mg

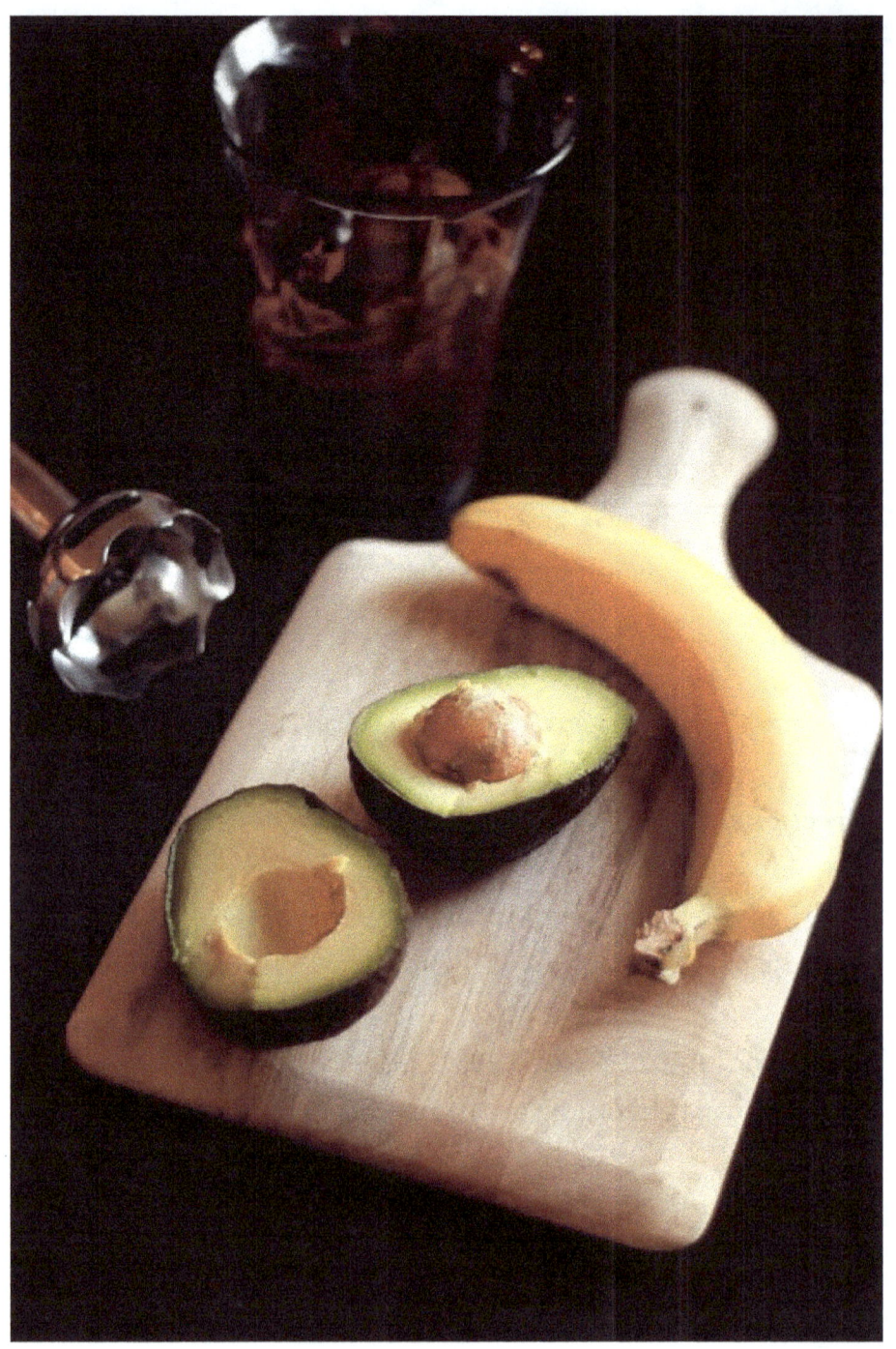

Banana Bars

Time To Prepare: ten minutes
Time to Cook: 60 minutes
Yield: Servings 4

Ingredients:
- ½ Cup Coconut Milk
- ½ Cup Melted Butter
- 1 Cup Chocolate Chips
- 1 Tsp. Baking Soda
- 1 Tsp. Pure Vanilla Extract
- 1/4 Tbsp. Cinnamon
- 2 Cup Brown Sugar
- 2 Cup Whole Wheat Flour
- 2 Eggs
- 5 Cup Ripe Mashed Banana
- Salt

Direction:
1. Preheat your oven to 170C.
2. Mix all together the ingredients to make the batter.
3. Put the batter in a wide tray and bake for about twenty minutes at 170C.
4. Serve with liquid chocolate or fruits.

Nutritional Info: ‖ Calories: 330 kcal ‖ Carbohydrates: 8.80 g ‖ Fat: 13.0 g ‖ Protein: 12.4 g.

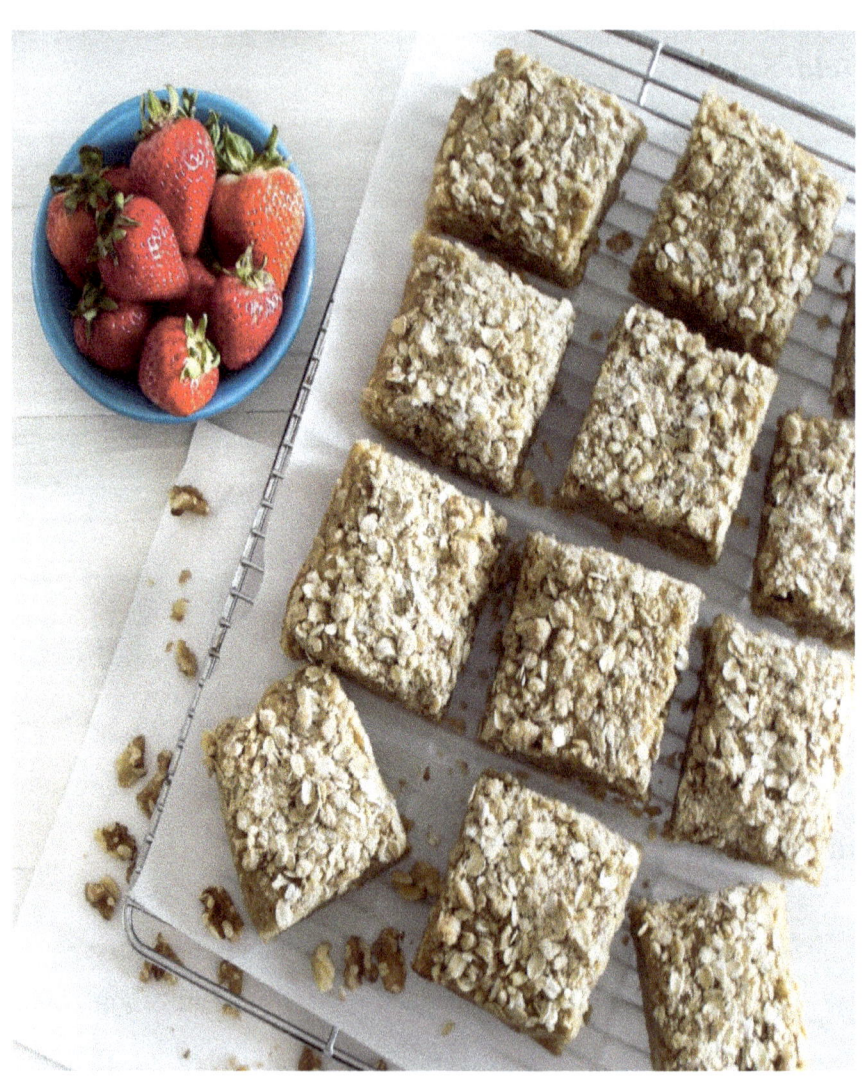

www.ingramcontent.com/pod-product-compliance
Lightning Source LLC
Chambersburg PA
CBHW070734030426
42336CB00013B/1975